This report contains the collective views of an international group of experts and does not necessarily represent the decisions or the stated policy of the United Nations Environment Programme, the International Labour Organisation, or the World Health Organization.

Environmental Health Criteria 217

Microbial Pest Control Agent

BACILLUS THURINGIENSIS

Published under the joint sponsorship of the United Nations Environment Programme, the International Labour Organisation, and the World Health Organization, and produced within the framework of the Inter-Organization Programme for the Sound Management of Chemicals.

World Health Organization
Geneva, 1999

The **International Programme on Chemical Safety (IPCS)**, established in 1980, is a joint venture of the United Nations Environment Programme (UNEP), the International Labour Organisation (ILO), and the World Health Organization (WHO). The overall objectives of the IPCS are to establish the scientific basis for assessment of the risk to human health and the environment from exposure to chemicals, through international peer review processes, as a prerequisite for the promotion of chemical safety, and to provide technical assistance in strengthening national capacities for the sound management of chemicals.

The **Inter-Organization Programme for the Sound Management of Chemicals (IOMC)** was established in 1995 by UNEP, ILO, the Food and Agriculture Organization of the United Nations, WHO, the United Nations Industrial Development Organization, the United Nations Institute for Training and Research, and the Organisation for Economic Co-operation and Development (Participating Organizations), following recommendations made by the 1992 UN Conference on Environment and Development to strengthen cooperation and increase coordination in the field of chemical safety. The purpose of the IOMC is to promote coordination of the policies and activities pursued by the Participating Organizations, jointly or separately, to achieve the sound management of chemicals in relation to human health and the environment.

WHO Library Cataloguing-in-Publication Data

Bacillus thuringiensis.

(Environmental health criteria ; 217)

1.Bacillus thuringinesis - pathogenicity 2.Pest control, Biological - methods 3.Insecticides - chemistry 4.Environmental exposure 5.Occupational exposure I.Series

ISBN 92 4 157217 5 (NLM Classification: QW 127.5.B2)
ISSN 0250-863X

The designations employed and the presentation of the material in this publication do not imply the expression of any opinion whatsoever on the part of the Secretariat of the World Health Organization concerning the legal status of any country, territory, city, or area or of its authorities, or concerning the delimitation of its frontiers or boundaries.

The mention of specific companies or of certain manufacturers' products does not imply that they are endorsed or recommended by the World Health Organization in preference to others of a similar nature that are not mentioned. Errors and omissions excepted, the names of proprietary products are distinguished by initial capital letters.

Printed in Finland
99/12798 – Vammala – 5000

CONTENTS

ENVIRONMENTAL HEALTH CRITERIA FOR *BACILLUS THURINGIENSIS*

PREAMBLE vii

ABBREVIATIONS xv

1. SUMMARY 1

1.1 Identity, biological characteristics, and analytical methods 1
1.2 Mode of action on target insects 2
1.3 Habitats 2
1.4 Commercial products, production and application . . . 3
1.5 Effects of Bt on non-target organisms 3
1.6 Exposure and effects of Bt on humans 4
1.7 Conclusions 4

2. IDENTITY, BIOLOGICAL PROPERTIES, AND ANALYTICAL METHODS 6

2.1 Identity 6
2.1.1 *Bacillus thuringiensis* (Bt) 6
2.1.2 Relationship between *Bacillus thuringiensis* and *Bacillus cereus* 6
2.1.3 Crystal composition and morphology 7
2.1.4 Classification of Bt subspecies 8
2.1.5 Genetics of ICP 10
2.1.6 Beta-exotoxin 14
2.1.7 Other Bt metabolites 17
2.2 Bioassays 18
2.2.1 Spore counts 18
2.2.2 International bioassay for ICPs 18

3. MODE OF ACTION ON TARGET INSECTS 19

3.1 Bioactivity of field isolates 19
3.2 Mechanism of action of Bt formulations 19

3.3. Resistance of insect populations 21

4. NATURAL AND TREATED HABITATS 23

4.1 Natural occurrence of Bt 23
4.1.1 Bt in insect hosts 23
4.1.2 Bt in soil 24
4.1.3 Bt on plant surfaces 24
4.2 Treated habitats 25
4.3 Environmental fate, distribution and movement 25
4.3.1 Distribution and fate of Bt in terrestrial habitats 26
4.3.1.1 Fate of Bt and ICP on plant surfaces 26
4.3.1.2 Fate of Bt in soil 27
4.3.2 Distribution and fate of Bt in aquatic habitats 29
4.3.3 Transport of Bt by non-target organisms . . . 30

5. COMMERCIAL PRODUCTION 31

5.1 History of Bt and its commercial applications 31
5.1.1 Production levels 31
5.1.2 Production processes, formulations and quality standards 31
5.1.3 General patterns of use 32
5.1.3.1 Applications in agriculture and forestry 32
5.1.3.2 Applications in vector control 34

6. EFFECTS ON ANIMALS 36

6.1 Mammals 36
6.1.1 Oral exposure 37
6.1.2 Inhalation exposure 39
6.1.3 Dermal exposure 39
6.1.4 Dermal scarification exposure 40
6.1.5 Subcutaneous inoculation 40
6.1.6 Ocular exposure 40
6.1.7 Intraperitoneal exposure 41
6.1.7.1 Immune-intact animals 43

6.1.7.2 Immune-suppressed animals 44
6.1.8 Effects of activated Bt ICP 45
6.1.9 Studies in wild animals 45
6.2 Effects on birds 45
6.3 Effects on aquatic vertebrates 47
6.4 Effects on invertebrates 49
6.4.1 Effects on invertebrates other than insects . 49
6.4.2 Effects on non-target insects 50
6.4.2.1 Aquatic insects 50
6.4.2.2 Terrestrial insects 54
6.4.2.3 Honey-bees 59
6.4.2.4 Parasitoids 60

7. EXPOSURE AND EFFECTS ON HUMANS 63

7.1 *Bacillus thuringiensis* 63
7.1.1 Experimental exposure of humans 63
7.1.2 Exposure of workers during manufacture .. 64
7.1.3 Exposure of workers in spraying operations 64
7.1.4 Exposure of human populations by spraying operations over populated areas. 65
7.1.5 Clinical case reports 65
7.1.6 Dietary exposure of the general population . 66
7.2 *Bacillus cereus* 67

8. EVALUATION OF HUMAN HEALTH RISKS AND EFFECTS ON THE ENVIRONMENT 69

9. CONCLUSIONS AND RECOMMENDATIONS 70

10. PREVIOUS EVALUATIONS BY INTERNATIONAL ORGANISATIONS 71

REFERENCES 72

RÉSUMÉ 94

RESUMEN 100

NOTE TO READERS OF THE CRITERIA MONOGRAPHS

Every effort has been made to present information in the criteria monographs as accurately as possible without unduly delaying their publication. In the interest of all users of the Environmental Health Criteria monographs, readers are requested to communicate any errors that may have occurred to the Director of the International Programme on Chemical Safety, World Health Organization, Geneva, Switzerland, in order that they may be included in corrigenda.

* * *

A detailed data profile and a legal file can be obtained from the International Register of Potentially Toxic Chemicals, Case postage 356, 1219 Châtelaine, Geneva, Switzerland (telephone no. + 41 22 – 9799111, fax no. + 41 22 – 7973460, E-mail irptc@unep.ch).

* * *

This publication was made possible by grant number 5 U01 ES02617-15 from the National Institute of Environmental Health Sciences, National Institutes of Health, USA, and by financial support from the European Commission.

Environmental Health Criteria

P R E A M B L E

Objectives

In 1973 the WHO Environmental Health Criteria Programme was initiated with the following objectives:

(i) to assess information on the relationship between exposure to environmental pollutants and human health, and to provide guidelines for setting exposure limits;

(ii) to identify new or potential pollutants;

(iii) to identify gaps in knowledge concerning the health effects of pollutants;

(iv) to promote the harmonization of toxicological and epidemiological methods in order to have internationally comparable results.

The first Environmental Health Criteria (EHC) monograph, on mercury, was published in 1976 and since that time an ever-increasing number of assessments of chemicals and of physical effects have been produced. In addition, many EHC monographs have been devoted to evaluating toxicological methodology, e.g., for genetic, neurotoxic, teratogenic and nephrotoxic effects. Other publications have been concerned with epidemiological guidelines, evaluation of short-term tests for carcinogens, biomarkers, effects on the elderly and so forth.

Since its inauguration the EHC Programme has widened its scope, and the importance of environmental effects, in addition to health effects, has been increasingly emphasized in the total evaluation of chemicals.

The original impetus for the Programme came from World Health Assembly resolutions and the recommendations of the 1972 UN Conference on the Human Environment. Subsequently the work became an integral part of the International Programme on Chemical Safety (IPCS), a cooperative programme of UNEP, ILO and WHO. In this manner, with the strong support of the new partners, the importance of occupational health and environmental effects was fully recognized. The EHC monographs have become widely established, used and recognized throughout the world.

The recommendations of the 1992 UN Conference on Environment and Development and the subsequent establishment of the Intergovernmental Forum on Chemical Safety with the priorities for action in the six programme areas of Chapter 19, Agenda 21, all lend further weight to the need for EHC assessments of the risks of chemicals.

Scope

The criteria monographs are intended to provide critical reviews on the effect on human health and the environment of chemicals and of combinations of chemicals and physical and biological agents. As such, they include and review studies that are of direct relevance for the evaluation. However, they do not describe *every* study carried out. Worldwide data are used and are quoted from original studies, not from abstracts or reviews. Both published and unpublished reports are considered and it is incumbent on the authors to assess all the articles cited in the references. Preference is always given to published data. Unpublished data are only used when relevant published data are absent or when they are pivotal to the risk assessment. A detailed policy statement is available that describes the procedures used for unpublished proprietary data so that this information can be used in the evaluation without compromising its confidential nature (WHO (1990) Revised Guidelines for the Preparation of Environmental Health Criteria Monographs. PCS/90.69, Geneva, World Health Organization).

In the evaluation of human health risks, sound human data, whenever available, are preferred to animal data. Animal and *in vitro* studies provide support and are used mainly to supply evidence missing from human studies. It is mandatory that research on human subjects is conducted in full accord with ethical principles, including the provisions of the Helsinki Declaration.

The EHC monographs are intended to assist national and international authorities in making risk assessments and subsequent risk management decisions. They represent a thorough evaluation of risks and are not, in any sense, recommendations for regulation or standard setting. These latter are the exclusive purview of national and regional governments.

Content

The layout of EHC monographs for chemicals is outlined below.

- Summary — a review of the salient facts and the risk evaluation of the chemical
- Identity — physical and chemical properties, analytical methods
- Sources of exposure
- Environmental transport, distribution and transformation
- Environmental levels and human exposure
- Kinetics and metabolism in laboratory animals and humans
- Effects on laboratory mammals and *in vitro* test systems
- Effects on humans
- Effects on other organisms in the laboratory and field
- Evaluation of human health risks and effects on the environment
- Conclusions and recommendations for protection of human health and the environment
- Further research
- Previous evaluations by international bodies, e.g., IARC, JECFA, JMPR

Selection of chemicals

Since the inception of the EHC Programme, the IPCS has organized meetings of scientists to establish lists of priority chemicals for subsequent evaluation. Such meetings have been held in: Ispra, Italy, 1980; Oxford, United Kingdom, 1984; Berlin, Germany, 1987; and North Carolina, USA, 1995. The selection of chemicals has been based on the following criteria: the existence of scientific evidence that the substance presents a hazard to human health and/or the environment; the possible use, persistence, accumulation or degradation of the substance shows that there may be significant human or environmental exposure; the size and nature of populations at risk (both human and other species) and risks for environment; international concern, i.e. the substance is of major interest to several countries; adequate data on the hazards are available.

If an EHC monograph is proposed for a chemical not on the priority list, the IPCS Secretariat consults with the Cooperating Organizations and all the Participating Institutions before embarking on the preparation of the monograph.

Procedures

The order of procedures that result in the publication of an EHC monograph is shown in the flow chart. A designated staff member of IPCS, responsible for the scientific quality of the document, serves as Responsible Officer (RO). The IPCS Editor is responsible for layout and language. The first draft, prepared by consultants or, more usually, staff from an IPCS Participating Institution, is based initially on data provided from the International Register of Potentially Toxic Chemicals, and reference data bases such as Medline and Toxline.

The draft document, when received by the RO, may require an initial review by a small panel of experts to determine its scientific quality and objectivity. Once the RO finds the document acceptable as a first draft, it is distributed, in its unedited form, to well over 150 EHC contact points throughout the world who are asked to comment on its completeness and accuracy and, where necessary, provide additional material. The contact points, usually designated by governments, may be Participating Institutions, IPCS Focal Points, or individual scientists known for their particular expertise. Generally some four months are allowed before the comments are considered by the RO and author(s). A second draft incorporating comments received and approved by the Director, IPCS, is then distributed to Task Group members, who carry out the peer review, at least six weeks before their meeting.

The Task Group members serve as individual scientists, not as representatives of any organization, government or industry. Their function is to evaluate the accuracy, significance and relevance of the information in the document and to assess the health and environmental risks from exposure to the chemical. A summary and recommendations for further research and improved safety aspects are also required. The composition of the Task Group is dictated by the range of expertise required for the subject of the meeting and by the need for a balanced geographical distribution.

EHC PREPARATION FLOW CHART

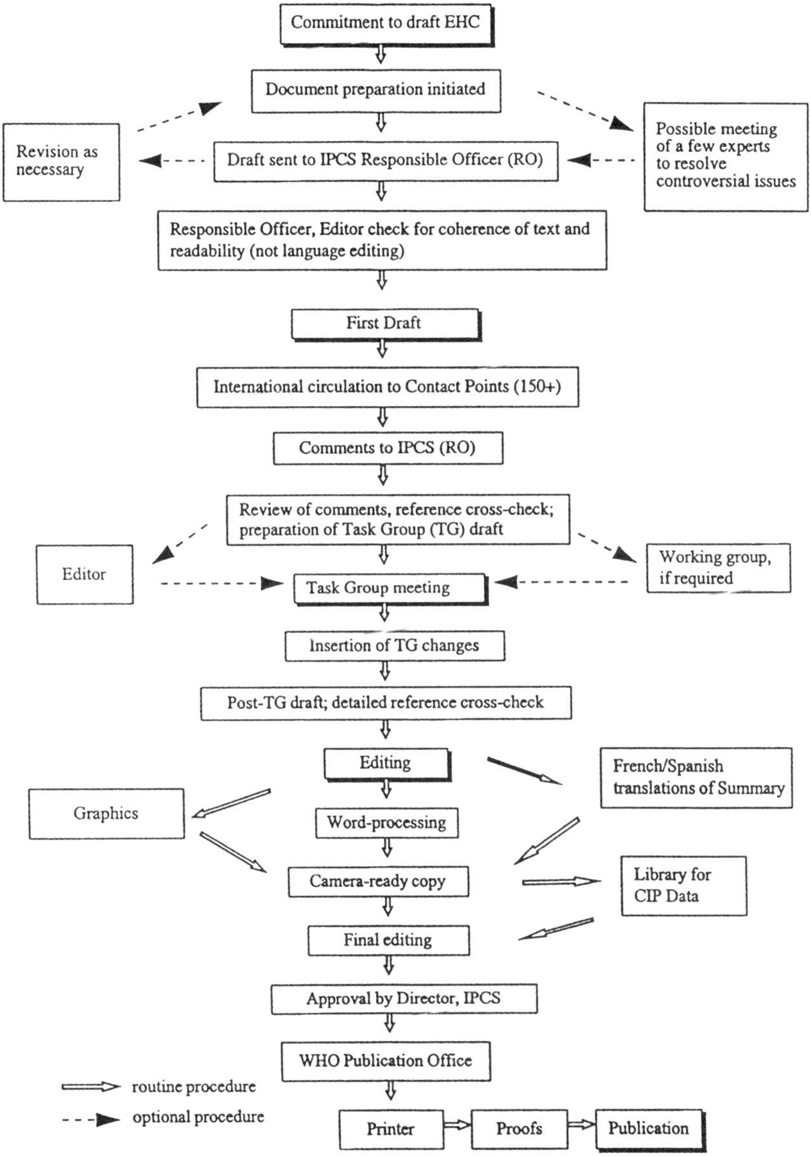

The three cooperating organizations of the IPCS recognize the important role played by nongovernmental organizations. Representatives from relevant national and international associations may be invited to join the Task Group as observers. While observers may provide a valuable contribution to the process, they can only speak at the invitation of the Chairperson. Observers do not participate in the final evaluation of the chemical; this is the sole responsibility of the Task Group members. When the Task Group considers it to be appropriate, it may meet *in camera*.

All individuals who as authors, consultants or advisers participate in the preparation of the EHC monograph must, in addition to serving in their personal capacity as scientists, inform the RO if at any time a conflict of interest, whether actual or potential, could be perceived in their work. They are required to sign a conflict of interest statement. Such a procedure ensures the transparency and probity of the process.

When the Task Group has completed its review and the RO is satisfied as to the scientific correctness and completeness of the document, it then goes for language editing, reference checking, and preparation of camera-ready copy. After approval by the Director, IPCS, the monograph is submitted to the WHO Office of Publications for printing. At this time a copy of the final draft is sent to the Chairperson and Rapporteur of the Task Group to check for any errors.

It is accepted that the following criteria should initiate the updating of an EHC monograph: new data are available that would substantially change the evaluation; there is public concern for health or environmental effects of the agent because of greater exposure; an appreciable time period has elapsed since the last evaluation.

All Participating Institutions are informed, through the EHC progress report, of the authors and institutions proposed for the drafting of the documents. A comprehensive file of all comments received on drafts of each EHC monograph is maintained and is available on request. The Chairpersons of Task Groups are briefed before each meeting on their role and responsibility in ensuring that these rules are followed.

WHO TASK GROUP ON ENVIRONMENTAL HEALTH CRITERIA FOR *BACILLUS THURINGIENSIS*

Members

Professor D. Calamari, Department of Biology, Structure and Function, University of Milan, Varese, Italy

Dr C. Cummins, Institute of Terrestrial Ecology, Monks Wood, Abbots Ripton, Huntingdon, Cambridgeshire, United Kingdom

Dr N. Gratz, Commugny, Switzerland (*Rapporteur*)

Dr A. Klier, Unité de Biochimie Microbienne, Département des Biotechnologies, Institut Pasteur, Paris, France

Professor P. Lüthy, Microbiological Institute ETH, Zurich, Switzerland

Dr C.M. Scanlan, Texas A & M University, Department of Veterinary Pathobiology, Texas Veterinary Medical Center, Texas, USA (*Chairman*)

Observers

Dr R.J. Cibulsky, Abbott Laboratories, Chemical and Agricultural Products, North Chicago, Illinois, USA

Dr E. Cozzi, Clinical Research and Development, Animal Health Products, Abbott Laboratories, North Chicago, Illinois, USA

Dr M. Ronchin, International Centre for Pesticide Safety, Busto Garolfo, Milan, Italy

Secretariat

Professor M. Maroni, International Centre for Pesticide Safety, Busto Garolfo, Milan, Italy

Dr R. Plestina, Zagreb, Croatia

ENVIRONMENTAL HEALTH CRITERIA FOR *BACILLUS THURINGIENSIS*

A WHO Task Group on Environmental Health Criteria for the microbial pest control agent *Bacillus thuringiensis* (Bt) met at the International Centre for Pesticide Safety in Busto Garolfo, Milan, Italy, from 27 to 31 October 1997. Professor M. Maroni, Director of the Centre, welcomed participants on behalf of the Centre, which was responsible for organizing the meeting. Dr R. Plestina, IPCS temporary adviser, opened the meeting and welcomed participants on behalf of Dr M. Mercier, Director of IPCS. The Group reviewed and revised the draft and made an evaluation of the risks for human health and the environment from exposure to Bt products. Drs R. Plestina and A. Aitio of the IPCS Central Unit were responsible for the scientific aspects of the monograph, and Dr P.G. Jenkins for the editing. The assistance of manufacturers, notably Abbott Laboratories, in providing unpublished documentation for the review is greatly appreciated.

Microbial Pest Control Agents (MPCAs), notably products of various Bt subspecies, are increasingly used in pest management programmes against the larvae of several insect pests of major agricultural crops and forests, and several insect vectors of human diseases, and some nuisance pests. Bt products have been used worldwide, and their commercial production is about 1% of that of chemical pesticides. A number of reviews have recently been published on various aspects of Bt (Entwistle et al., 1983; McClintock et al., 1995; Cannon, 1996; Dean et al., 1996; Kumar et al., 1996; Schnepf et al., 1998; Nielsen-LeRoux et al., 1998).

The activities in preparing this document were recommended by an Informal Consultation on the Safety of Microbial Pest Control Agents held in Geneva in June 1993. The first draft of the monograph was prepared by a drafting group in 1994 and was subsequently amended by Professor C.M. Scanlan (Texas A&M University, Department of Veterinary Pathobiology, The Texas Veterinary Medical Center, Texas, USA). The revised draft was circulated to the IPCS contact points. Based on the comments received, it was amended and updated by Drs B.M. Hansen and N.B. Hendriksen (National Environmental Research Institute, Roskilde, Denmark). The document was finally approved by the Task Group members.

ABBREVIATIONS

Bc	*Bacillus cereus*
Bt	*Bacillus thuringiensis*
Bta	*Bacillus thuringiensis* subspecies *aizawai*
Btd	*Bacillus thuringiensis* subspecies *darmstadiensis*
Bte	*Bacillus thuringiensis* subspecies *entomocidus*
Btg	*Bacillus thuringiensis* subspecies *galleriae*
Bti	*Bacillus thuringiensis* subspecies *israelensis*
Btk	*Bacillus thuringiensis* subspecies *kurstaki*
Btko	*Bacillus thuringiensis* subspecies *konkukian*
Btt	*Bacillus thuringiensis* subspecies *thuringiensis*
Btte	*Bacillus thuringiensis* subspecies *tenebrionis*
cfu	colony forming unit
GILSP	good industrial large-scale practice
GMO	genetically modified organism
HPLC	high-performance liquid chromatography
ICP	insecticidal crystal protein
ITU	international toxic unit
IUPAC	International Union of Pure and Applied Chemistry
MPCA	microbial pest control agent
NTO	non-target organism
PCR	polymerase chain reaction
SDS-PAGE	sodium dodecyl sulfate polyacrylamide gel electrophoresis

1. SUMMARY

This monograph deals with microbial pest control agents (MCPAs) based on *Bacillus thuringiensis* (Bt). This bacterium is also a key source of genes for transgenic expression to provide pest resistance in plants and microorganisms as pest control agents in so-called genetically modified organisms (GMOs). The potential effects on human health and the environment of GMOs involve several aspects that are only remotely or not at all related to Bt products, and they are therefore outside the scope of this monograph.

1.1 Identity, biological characteristics and analytical methods

Bt is a facultative anaerobic, gram-positive bacterium that forms characteristic protein inclusions adjacent to the endospore. Bt subspecies can synthesize more than one parasporal inclusion. Bt is genetically indistinguishable from Bc, except for the ability of Bt to produce parasporal crystalline inclusions, which are toxic for certain invertebrates, especially species of insect larvae belonging to the insect orders *Coleoptera*, *Diptera* and *Lepidoptera*. The parasporal inclusions are formed by different insecticidal crystal proteins (ICP). The crystals have various shapes (bipyramidal, cuboidal, flat rhomboid, spherical or composite with two crystal types), depending on their ICP composition. A partial correlation between crystal morphology, ICP composition, and bioactivity against target insects has been established.

The basic phenotypic taxon is the subspecies, identified by the flagellar (H) serotype. By 1998, 67 subspecies had been described. The genes that encode the ICPs are mostly on plasmids. Each ICP is the product of a single gene. Most plasmids with ICP genes are readily transferred by conjugation between Bt strains and may be transferred to related species of bacteria. The phenotypic classification has now been complemented by molecular biological characterization, based on the sequence of the crystal (*cry* and *cyt*) genes rather than target organism specificity. Different domains of the ICP are responsible for host susceptibility (receptor recognition) and toxicity (pore formation).

Techniques commonly used to characterize Bt strains or the ICP itself include cell wall fatty acid analysis, monoclonal antibodies, oligonucleotide DNA probes, plasmid profiles, polymerase chain reaction (PCR) analysis, DNA fingerprinting and SDS-PAGE profiles.

Beta-exotoxin, a heat-stable nucleotide, is produced by some Bt subspecies during vegetative growth and may contaminate the products. Beta-exotoxin is toxic for almost all forms of life including humans and the target insect orders. During vegetative growth, various Bt strains produce an assortment of antibiotics, enzymes, metabolites and toxins, including Bc toxins, that may have detrimental effects on both target organisms and non-target organisms (NTOs). Spore counts do not accurately reflect the insecticidal activity of a Bt strain or Bt product. The potency (ITU/mg) of each Bt product is bioassayed using an international standard that uses a specific test insect.

1.2 Mode of action on target insects

The sporulated Bt with ICP or spore-ICP complexes must be ingested by a susceptible insect larva. The efficacy of the ICP depends on the solubilization in the midgut, the conversion of the protoxin to the biologically active toxin by proteolytic enzymes, specific membrane receptor binding by the C-terminal domain of the active toxin, and pore formation by the N-terminal domain with subsequent lysis of the epithelial cells. Spore germination and proliferation of the vegetative cells into the haemocoel may result in a septicaemia, contributing to the cause of death. Receptor binding by the ICP is the major determinant of host specificity by the different Bt ICPs.

1.3 Habitats

Many different Bt subspecies have been isolated from dead or dying insects mostly from the orders *Coleoptera*, *Diptera* and *Lepidoptera*, but many subspecies have also been isolated from soil, leaf surfaces and other habitats. The carcasses of dead insects often contain large quantities of spores and ICPs that may enter the environment. The coleopteran-active and lepidopteran-active Bt subspecies are primarily associated with the soil and phylloplane (leaf surfaces), whereas the dipteran-active Bt subspecies are commonly found in aquatic environments. In the environment, the spores persist and vegetative growth may occur when conditions are favourable and nutrients are available.

1.4 Commercial products, production and application

Conventional Bt products, which utilize naturally-occurring Bt strains, account for approximately 90% of the world MPCA market. Most Bt products contain ICP and viable spores, but in some Bti products the spores are inactivated. Each year some 13 000 tonnes are produced using aerobic fermentation technology. Conventional Bt products have been targeted primarily against lepidopteran pests of agricultural and forestry crops; however in recent years, Bt strains active against coleopteran pests have also been marketed. Strains of Bti active against dipteran vectors of parasitic and viral diseases are being used in public health programmes.

Commercial Bt formulations may be applied as an insecticide to foliage, soil, water environments or food storage facilities. After the application of a Bt subspecies to an ecosystem, the vegetative cells and spores may persist at gradually decreasing concentrations for weeks, months or years as a component of the natural microflora. The ICPs, however, are rendered biologically inactive within hours or days.

1.5 Effects of Bt on non-target organisms

Studies on mammals, particularly those on laboratory animals, have evaluated possible infectivity and toxicity of various Bt preparations, which include the ICPs, vegetative cells and spores. The ICPs, spores and vegetative cells of the Bt subspecies, which were administered by different routes, were mostly non-pathogenic and non-toxic to the various animal species tested. The vegetative cells and/or spores of Bt were demonstrated to persist for weeks without causing adverse effects. Bt has not been observed to adversely affect birds, fish or many other non-target aquatic vertebrates tested in a large number of laboratory and field studies. Relatively few species of aquatic invertebrates are susceptible to Bt under either laboratory or field conditions. Bt does not adversely affect earthworms.

The Bt subspecies have generally been shown to be highly specific in their insecticidal activity for *Coleoptera*, *Diptera* and *Lepidoptera* and have demonstrated little, if any, direct toxicity to non-target arthropods. Most of the existing safety data on non-target arthropods has been generated using the Bt subspecies with activity against *Diptera* and *Lepidoptera*.

Studies of Bti formulations free of toxic contaminants have not demonstrated deleterious effects on the vast majority of non-target arthropods. Some midges (*Diptera*: *Chironomidae*), which are closely related to mosquitos, have been shown to be susceptible to high dosages of Bti, but are not affected by mosquito larvicidal dosages. In field studies, transient decreases or increases in populations of some non-target arthropods have been reported.

Many insect orders have been tested in either the laboratory or field, most of which have shown no effect from Btk.

Mortality has been observed in honey-bees (*Apis mellifera*) after exposure to vegetatively growing Btt and Btk, but the effect does not seem to be related to spores or ICPs. In laboratory and field studies Btg demonstrated no adverse effect on honey-bees.

Bte strains that produce beta-exotoxin have been shown to have adverse effects on non-target arthropods.

1.6 Exposure and effects of Bt on humans

The field application of Bt products can result in considerable aerosol and dermal exposure of workers. Agricultural uses of Bt can result in Bt contamination of potable water and food. With the exception of case reports on ocular and dermal irritation, no adverse health effects have been documented after occupational exposure to Bt products. Human volunteers ingested and inhaled large quantities of a Btk formulation but experienced no adverse health effects. Antibody titres to the vegetative cells, spores and spore-crystal complexes have been demonstrated in workers who spray Bt products; however, no adverse health effects were reported. There have been some case reports on the occurrence of Bt in patients with different infectious diseases. However, none of these studies unequivocally demonstrates an actual risk to human health from the use of Bt. Bt has not been reported to cause adverse effects on human health when present in drinking-water or food.

1.7 Conclusions

Owing to their specific mode of action, Bt products are unlikely to pose any hazard to humans or other vertebrates or to the great majority of non-target invertebrates provided that they are free from non-Bt microorganisms and biologically active products other than the ICPs. Bt products may be safely used for the control of insect pests of agricultural and horticultural crops as well as forests. They are also safe for use in aquatic environments including drinking-water reservoirs for the control of mosquito, black fly and nuisance insect larvae. However, it should be noted that vegetative Bt has the potential for the production of Bc-like toxins, the significance of which as a cause of human disease is not known.

2. IDENTITY, BIOLOGICAL PROPERTIES, AND ANALYTICAL METHODS

2.1 Identity

Commercial *Bacillus thuringiensis* (Bt) products are microbial pest control agents (MPCAs) containing specific insecticidal crystalline proteins (ICPs) and most often living spores as well as formulating agents. They are processed fermentation products.

2.1.1 Bacillus thuringiensis

Bt is a facultative anaerobic, motile, gram-positive, spore-forming bacterium. The formation of parasporal crystals adjacent to the endospore during sporulation stages III to IV distinguishes Bt from other *Bacillus* species.

Bt, like other *Bacillus* species, has been classified on the basis of its cellular, cultural, biochemical and genetic characteristics (Baumann et al., 1984; Claus & Berkley, 1986; Slepecky & Hemphill, 1992; Carlson & Kolstø, 1993; Hansen et al., 1998). In 1958, Heimpel & Angus (1958) introduced a classification scheme to identify these crystalliferous bacteria based on their morphological and biochemical characteristics. However recent molecular analysis shows that several variations can be found within serotypes, and that specific biochemical characteristics do not always refer to a specific serotype (Helgason et al., 1998; Hansen et al., 1998).

2.1.2 Relationship between **Bacillus thuringiensis** *and* **Bacillus cereus**

Bt is a member of the Bc group, which also contains *Bacillus cereus* (Bc), *B. mycoides* and *B. anthracis*. Furthermore, the psychrotolerant *B. weihenstephanensis* has recently been proposed as a new member of the group (Lechner et al., 1998). Bt can only be distinguished from Bc by the production during the sporulation process of one or more inclusion bodies, which have been found to be toxic for invertebrates, primarily insect species in the orders *Coleoptera*, *Diptera* and *Lepidoptera* (de Barjac, 1981b; Andrews et al., 1987). Several studies have been dedicated to a comparison of Bt and Bc on the basis of characters not related to the production of ICPs (Hendriksen & Hansen, 1998). Phenotypic differentiation of Bt and Bc is not possible on the basis of morphology or utilization of organic compounds (Baumann et al., 1984; Logan & Berkeley, 1984; Priest et al., 1988), characterization of cell content of fatty acids (Väisänen et al., 1991) or sugars (Wunschel et al., 1994), multilocus enzyme electrophoresis (Zahner et al., 1989; Carlson et al., 1994), enterotoxin production (Damgaard et al., 1996a; Hansen & Hendriksen, 1997a), or serological- and phage-typing techniques (Ohba & Aizawa, 1978; 1986; Väisänen et al., 1991; Murakami et al., 1993; Ahmed et al., 1995). Likewise, genotypic differentiation of Bt and Bc is not possible by DNA homology analysis (Kaneko et al., 1978), ribotyping (Priest et al., 1994; Demezas & Bell, 1995), 16S rDNA sequencing (Ash et al., 1991); analysis of the 16S-23S internal transcribed sequence (Wunschel et al., 1994; Bourque et al., 1995), PCR analysis of genes encoding Bc-like toxic products (Damgaard et al., 1996b; Asano et al., 1997; Hansen & Hendriksen, 1997b) or pulsed field gel electrophoresis (Carlson & Kolstø, 1993; Carlson et al., 1994). Giffel et al. (1997) found differences in 16S rDNA sequences between a limited number Bt and Bc. Beattie et al. (1998) were able to discriminate among members of the Bc group by Fourier transform infrared spectroscopy, and Brousseau et al. (1992) were able to distinguish Bt and Bc by random amplified polymorphic DNA fingerprinting. However, the transfer of ICP encoding plasmids from Bt to Bc makes the receptor Bc indistinguishable from Bt, and vice versa (González et al., 1981, 1982).

2.1.3 *Crystal composition and morphology*

The existence of parasporal inclusions in Bt was first noted in 1915 (Berliner, 1915), but their protein composition was not delineated until the 1950s (Angus, 1954). Hannay (1953) detected the crystalline fine structure that is a property of most of the parasporal inclusions. Bt subspecies can synthesize more than one inclusion, which may contain different ICPs. ICPs have also been called delta endotoxins; however, since the term endotoxin usually refers to toxins associated with the outer membranes of gram-negative bacteria, comprising a core lipopoplysaccharide, lipid A and somatic (O) antigens, this term is not used in this monograph. Depending on their ICP composition, the crystals have various forms (bipyramidal, cuboidal, flat rhomboid, or a composite with two or more crystal types). A partial correlation between crystal morphology, ICP composition, and bioactivity against target insects has been established

(Bulla et al., 1977; Höfte & Whiteley, 1989; Lynch & Baumann, 1985).

2.1.4 Classification of Bt subspecies

The classification of Bt subspecies based on the serological analysis of the flagella (H) antigens was introduced in the early 1960s (de Barjac & Bonnefoi, 1962). This classification by serotype has been supplemented by morphological and biochemical criteria (de Barjac, 1981a). Until 1977, only 13 Bt subspecies had been described, and at that time all subspecies were toxic to Lepidopteran larvae only. The discovery of other subspecies toxic to *Diptera* (Goldberg & Margalit, 1977), *Coleoptera* (Krieg et al., 1983) and apparently *Nematoda* (Narva et al., 1991) enlarged the host range and markedly increased the number of subspecies. Up to the end of 1998, over 67 subspecies based on flagellar H-serovars had been identified (Table 1). Updated lists of the serovarieties can be obtained from the reference centre of the Pasteur Institute in Paris (Unité des Bactéries Entomopathogènes, Institut Pasteur, Paris, France).

Table 1. Current classification of 67 *Bacillus thuringiensis* subspecies based on their flagellar (H) antigens[a]

Flagellar antigens	*B. thuringiensis* subspecies	Flagellar antigens	*B. thuringiensis* subspecies
1	*thuringiensis*	28a, 28c	*jegathesan*
2	*finitimus*	29	*amagiensis*
3a, 3c	*alesti*	30	*medellin*
3a, 3b, 3c	*kurstaki*	31	*toguchini*
3a, 3d	*sumiyoshiensis*	32	*cameroun*
3a, 3d, 3e	*fukuokaensis*	33	*leesis*
4a, 4b	*sotto*	34	*konkukian*
4a, 4c	*kenyae*	35	*seoulensis*
5a, 5c	*galleriae*	36	*malaysiensis*
5a, 5c	*canadensis*	37	*anadalousiensis*
6	*entomocidus*	38	*oswaldocruzi*
7	*aizawai*	39	*brasiliensis*
8a, 8b	*morrisoni*	40	*huazhongensis*
8a, 8c	*ostriniae*	41	*sooncheon*

Table 1 (contd).

Flagellar antigens	*B. thuringiensis* subspecies	Flagellar antigens	*B. thuringiensis* subspecies
8b, 8d	*nigeriensis*	42	*jinghongiensis*
9	*tolworthi*	43	*guiyanguebsus*
10a, 10b	*darmstadiensis*	44	*higo*
10a, 10c	*londrina*	45	*roskildiensis*
11a, 11b	*toumanoffi*	46	*chanpaisis*
11a, 11c	*kyushuensis*	47	*wratislaviensis*
12	*thompsoni*	48	*balearica*
13	*pakistani*	49	*muju*
14	*israelensis*	50	*navarrensis*
15	*dakota*	51	*xiaguangiensis*
16	*indiana*	52	*kim*
17	*tohokuensis*	53	*asturiensis*
18a, 18b	*kumamotoensis*	54	*poloniensis*
18a, 18c	*yosoo*	55	*palmanyolensis*
19	*tochigiensis*	56	*rongseni*
20a, 20b	*yunnanensis*	57	*pirenaica*
20a, 20c	*pondicheriensis*	58	*argentinensis*
21	*colmeri*	59	*iberica*
22	*shandongiensis*	60	*pingluonsis*
23	*japonensis*	61	*sylvestriensis*
24a, 24b	*neoleonensis*	62	*zhaodongensis*
24a, 24c	*novosibirsk*	63	*bolivia*
25	*coreanensis*	64	*azorensis*
26	*silo*	65	*pulsiensis*
27	*mexicanensis*	66	*gracioensis*
28a, 28b	*monterrey*	67	*vazensis*

[a] Data provided by the Unité des Bactéries Entomopathogènes, Institut Pasteur, Paris, France

Crystal serology has shown that a particular crystal type may be produced by more than one H-serovar (Krywienczyk et al., 1978; Smith, 1987).

2.1.5 Genetics of ICP

In the early 1980s, it was established that most genes coding for the ICPs reside on large transmissible plasmids, of which most are readily exchanged between strains by conjugation (González & Carlton, 1980; González et al., 1981). Since these initial studies, numerous ICP genes have been cloned, sequenced and used to construct Bt strains with novel insecticidal spectra (Höfte & Whiteley, 1989).

The currently known crystal (*cry*) gene types encode ICPs that are specific to either *Lepidoptera* (*cryI*), *Diptera* and *Lepidoptera* (*cryII*), *Coleoptera* (*cryIII*), *Diptera* (*cryIV*), or *Coleoptera* and *Lepidoptera* (*cryV*) (Höfte & Whiteley, 1989). A separate designation is used for the cytolytic (*cyt*) genes that encode a nonspecific cytolytic factor, present in Bti ICP and some other Bt subspecies. However, due to the increasing number of characterized ICP genes and inconsistencies in the existing *cry* gene nomenclature, which is based on insecticidal spectrum, Crickmore et al. (1998) proposed a new nomenclature based on ICP gene sequences. The new *cry* genes are listed in Tables 2 and 3, and Table 4 is a conversion list from old to new *cry* gene names. Current identification of Bt employs both the identity of the *cry* genes, which define the host range, and the H-serovars, which define the subspecies, and recently DNA fingerprinting has been used for further characterization of subspecies (Hansen et al., 1998).

The ICP gene sequences provided the basis for the construction of gene-specific probes to screen established Bt strains by hybridization and PCR analysis for the presence of known nucleotide sequences, and for characterizing the ICPs from new Bt isolates (Prefontaine et al., 1987; Juarez-Perez et al., 1997; Bravo et al., 1998; Shevelev et al., 1998). These studies have permitted the distinction of numerous subclasses of ICP genes based on sequence homology and toxicity spectra of the encoded proteins.

All ICPs described to date attack the insect gut upon ingestion (see chapter 3). To date, each of the proteolytically activated ICP molecules with insecticidal activity has a variable C-terminal domain, which is responsible for receptor recognition (host susceptibility), and a conserved N-terminal domain, which induces pore formation (toxicity) (Li et al., 1991).

Table 2. *Bacillus thuringiensis* crystal protein genes (Crickmore et al., 1998)

Name	Acc No	Reference	Journal	Coding
Cry1aa1	M11250	Schnepf et al., 1985	JBC 260 6264-6272	527-4054
Cry1aa2	M10917	Shibano et al., 1985	Gene 34 243-251	153->2955
Cry1aa3	D00348	Shimizu et al., 1988	ABC 52 1565-1573	73-3603
Cry1aa4	X13535	Masson et al., 1989	NAR 17 446-446	1-3528
Cry1aa5	D17518	Udayasuriyan et al., 1994	BBB 58 830-835	81-3611
Cry1aa6	U43605	Masson et al., 1994	Mol Micro 14 851-860	1->1860
Cry1aa7	AF081790	Osman, 1998	unpublished	
Cry1aa8	I26149	Liu, 1996	USP 5556784	148-3675
Cry1ab1	M13898	Wabiko et al., 1986	DNA 5 305-314	142-3606
Cry1ab2	M12661	Thorne et al., 1986	J Bact 166 801-811	155-3625
Cry1ab3	M15271	Geiser et al., 1986	Gene 48 109-118	156-3623
Cry1ab4	D00117	Kondo et al., 1987	ABC 51 455-463	163-3630
Cry1ab5	X04698	Hofte et al., 1986	EJB 161 273-280	141-3605
Cry1ab6	M37263	Hefford et al., 1987	J Biotech 6 307-322	73-3540
Cry1ab7	X13233	Haider & Ellar, 1988	NAR 16 10927-10927	1-3465
Cry1ab8	M16463	Oeda et al., 1987	Gene 53 113-119	157-3624
Cry1ab9	X54939	Chak & Jen, 1993	PNSCRC 17 7-14	73-3540
Cry1ab10	A29125	Fischhoff et al., 1987	Bio/technology 5 807-813	peptide seq
Cry1ab11	I12419	Ely & Tippett, 1995	USP 5424409	73-
Cry1ab12	AF057670	Silva-Werneck et al., 1998	unpublished	41-3505
Cry1ac1	M11068	Adang et al., 1985	Gene 36 289-300	388-3921
Cry1ac2	M35524	Von Tersch et al., 1991	AEM 57 349-358	239-3772
Cry1ac3	X54159	Dardenne et al., 1990	NAR 18 5546-5546	339->2192
Cry1ac4	M73249	Payne et al., 1991	USP 4990332	1-3537
Cry1ac5	M73248	Payne et al., 1992	USP 5135867	1-3534
Cry1ac6	U43606	Masson et al., 1994	Mol Micro 14 851-860	1->1821
Cry1ac7	U87793	Herrera et al., 1994	AEM 60 682-690	976-4512
Cry1ac8	U87397	Omolo et al., 1997	Curr Micro 34 118-121	153-3686
Cry1ac9	U89872	Gleave et al., 1992	NZJCHS 20 27-36	388-3921
Cry1ac10	AJ002514	Sun & Yu, 1997	unpublished	388-3921
Cry1ac11	AJ130970	Makhdoom & Riazuddin, 1998	unpublished	156-3689
Cry1ac12	I12418	Ely & Tippett, 1995	USP 5424409	81->2990
Cry1ad1	M73250	Payne & Sick, 1993	USP 5246852	1-3537
Cry1ad2	A27531	Payne & Sick, 1995	AUP 632335	1-3537
Cry1ae1	M65252	Lee & Aronson, 1991	J Bact 173 6635-6638	81-3623
Cry1af1	U82003	Kang et al., 1997	unpublished	172->2905
Cry1ag1	AF081248	Osman, 1998	unpublished	
Cry1ba1	X06711	Brizzard & Whiteley, 1988	NAR 16 2723-2724	1-3684
Cry1ba2	X95704	Soetaert, 1996	unpublished	186-3869
Cry1bb1	L32020	Donovan et al., 1994	USP 5322687	67-3753
Cry1bc1	Z46442	Bishop et al., 1994	unpublished	141-3839
Cry1bd1	U70726	Kuo & Chak, 1999	unpublished	842-4534
Cry1be1		Payne et al., 1998	USP 5723758	1-3681
Cry1ca1	X07518	Honee et al., 1988	NAR 16 6240-6240	47-3613
Cry1ca2	X13620	Sanchis et al., 1989	Mol Micro 3 229-238	241->2711
Cry1ca3	M73251	Payne & Sick, 1993	USP 5246852	1-3570
Cry1ca4	A27642	Van Mellaert et al., 1990	EP 0400246	234-3800
Cry1ca5	X96682	Strizhov, 1996	unpublished	1->2286
Cry1cb1	M97880	Kalman et al., 1993	AEM 59 1131-1137	296-3823
Cry1da1	X54160	Hofte et al., 1990	NAR 18 5545-5545	264-3758

Table 2 (contd).

Name	Acc No	Reference	Journal	Coding
Cry1da2	I76415	Payne & Sick, 1997	USP 5691308	1-3495
Cry1db1	Z22511	Lambert, 1993	unpublished	241-3720
Cry1ea1	X53985	Visser et al., 1990	J Bact 172 6783-6788	130-3642
Cry1ea2	X56144	Bosse et al., 1990	NAR 18 7443-7443	1-3516
Cry1ea3	M73252	Payne & Sick, 1991	USP 5039523	1-3516
Cry1ea4	U94323	Barboza-Corona et al., 1998	WJMB 14 437-441	388-3900
Cry1ea5	A15535	Botterman et al., 1994	EP 0358557	54-3566
Cry1eb1	M73253	Payne & Sick, 1993	USP 5206166	1-3522
Cry1fa1	M63897	Chambers et al., 1991	J Bact 173 3966-3976	478-3999
Cry1fa2	M73254	Payne & Sick, 1993	USP 5188960	1-3525
Cry1fb1	Z22512	Lambert, 1993	unpublished	483-4004
Cry1fb2	AB012288	Masuda & Asano, 1998	unpublished	84-3587
Cry1fb3	AF062350	Song & Zhang, 1998	unpublished	
Cry1fb4	I73895	Payne et al., 1997	USP 5686069	peptide seq
Cry1ga1	Z22510	Lambert, 1993	unpublished	67-3564
Cry1ga2	Y09326	Shevelev et al., 1997	Febs Lett 404 148-152	692-4210
Cry1gb1	U70725	Kuo & Chak, 1999	unpublished	532-4038
Cry1ha1	Z22513	Lambert, 1993	unpublished	530-4045
Cry1hb1	U35780	Koo et al., 1995	unpublished	728-4195
Cry1ia1	X62821	Tailor et al., 1992	Mol Micro 6 1211-1217	355-2511
Cry1ia2	M98544	Gleave et al., 1993	AEM 59 1683-1687	1-2160
Cry1ia3	L36338	Shin et al., 1995	AEM 61 2402-2407	279-2438
Cry1ia4	L49391	Kostichka et al., 1996	J Bact 178 2141-2144	61-2217
Cry1ia5	Y08920	Selvapandiyan, 1996	unpublished	524-2680
Cry1ia6	AF076953	Zhong et al., 1998	unpublished	1-2157
Cry1ib1	U07642	Shin et al., 1995	AEM 61 2402-2407	237-2393
Cry1ic1	AF056933	Osman et al., 1998	unpublished	1-2157
Cry1i-like	I90732	Payne et al., 1998	See Table 3	peptide seq
Cry1ja1	L32019	Donovan et al., 1994	USP 5322687	99-3519
Cry1jb1	U31527	Von Tersch & Gonzalez, 1994	USP 5356623	177-3686
Cry1jc1	I90730	Payne et al., 1998	USP 5723758	peptide seq
Cry1ka1	U28801	Koo et al., 1995	FEMS 134 159-164	451-4098
Cry1-like	I90729	Payne et al., 1998	See Table 3	peptide seq
Cry2aa1	M31738	Donovan et al., 1989	JBC 264 4740-4740	156-2054
Cry2aa2	M23723	Widner & Whiteley, 1989	J Bact 171 965-974	1840-3741
Cry2aa3	D86064	Sasaki et al., 1997	Curr Micro 35 1-8	2007-3911
Cry2aa4	AF047038	Misra et al., 1998	Unpublished	10-1908
Cry2aa5	AJ132464	Yu & Pang, 1999	Unpublished	<1-1860
Cry2aa6	AJ132465	Yu & Pang , 1999	Unpublished	<1-1860
Cry2aa7	AJ132463	Yu & Pang, 1999	Unpublished	<1->1611
Cry2ab1	M23724	Widner & Whiteley, 1989	J Bact 171 965-974	1-1899
Cry2ab2	X55416	Dankocsik et al., 1990	Mol Micro 4 2087-2094	874-2775
Cry2ac1	X57252	Wu et al., 1991	FEMS 81 31-36	2125-3990
Cry3aa1	M22472	Hermstadt et al., 1987	Gene 57 37-46	25-1956
Cry3aa2	J02978	Sekar et al., 1987	PNAS 84 7036-7040	241-2175
Cry3aa3	Y00420	Hofte et al., 1987	NAR 15 7183-7183	566-2497
Cry3aa4	M30503	McPherson et al., 1988	Bio/technology 6 61-66	201-2135
Cry3aa5	M37207	Donovan et al., 1988	MGG 214 365-372	569-2503
Cry3aa6	U10985	Adams et al., 1994	Mol Micro 14 381-389	569-2503
Cry3ba1	X17123	Sick et al., 1990	NAR 18 1305-1305	25-1977

Table 2 (contd).

Name	Acc No	Reference	Journal	Coding
Cry3ba2	A07234	Peferoen et al., 1990	EP 0382990	342-2297
Cry3bb1	M89794	Donovan et al., 1992	AEM 58 3921-3927	202-2157
Cry3bb2	U31633	Donovan et al., 1995	USP 5378625	144-2099
Cry3bb3	I15475	Peferoen et al., 1995	USP 5466597	<1->1291
Cry3ca1	X59797	Lambert et al., 1992	Gene 110 131-132	232-2178
Cry4aa1	Y00423	Ward & Ellar, 1987	NAR 15 7195-7195	1-3540
Cry4aa2	D00248	Sen et al., 1988	ABC 52 873-878	393-3935
Cry4ba1	X07423	Chungjatpornchai et al., 1988	EJB 173 9-16	157-3564
Cry4ba2	X07082	Tungpradubkul et al., 1988	NAR 16 1637-1638	151-3558
Cry4ba3	M20242	Yamamoto et al., 1988	Gene 66 107-120	526-3933
Cry4ba4	D00247	Sen et al., 1988	ABC 52 873-878	461-3868
Cry5aa1	L07025	Sick et al., 1994	USP 5281530	1-4155
Cry5ab1	L07026	Narva et al., 1991	EP 0462721	1-3867
Cry5ac1	I34543	Payne et al., 1997	USP 5596071	1-3660
Cry5ba1	U19725	Payne et al., 1997	USP 5596071	1-3735
Cry6aa1	L07022	Narva et al., 1993	USP 5236843	1-1425
Cry6ba1	L07024	Narva et al., 1991	EP 0462721	1-1185
Cry7aa1	M64478	Lambert et al., 1992	AEM 58 2536-2542	184-3597
Cry7ab1	U04367	Payne & Fu, 1994	USP 5286486	1-3414
Cry7ab2	U04368	Payne & Fu, 1994	USP 5286486	1-3414
Cry8aa1	U04364	Foncerrada et al., 1992	EP 0498537	1-3471
Cry8ba1	U04365	Michaels et al., 1993	WO 93/15206	1-3507
Cry8ca1	U04366	Ogiwara et al., 1995	Curr Micro 30 227-235	1-3447
Cry9aa1	X58120	Smulevitch et al., 1991	FEBS 293 25-28	5807-9274
Cry9aa2	X58534	Gleave et al., 1992	JGM 138 55-62	385->3837
Cry9ba1	X75019	Shevelev et al., 1993	FEBS 336 79-82	26-3488
Cry9ca1	Z37527	Lambert et al., 1996	AEM 62 80-86	2096-5569
Cry9da1	D85560	Asano et al., 1997	AEM 63 1054-1057	47-3553
Cry9Da2	AF042733	Wasano & Ohba, 1998	Unpublished	<1->1937
Cry9Ea1	AB011496	Midoh & Oyama, 1998	Unpublished	211-3660
Cry9 like	AF093107	Wasano & Ohba, 1998	See Table 3	<1->1917
Cry10Aa1	M12662	Thorne et al., 1986	J Bact 166 801-811	941-2965
Cry10Aa2	E00614	Uorufuiirudo, 1996	JP 1986005098	940-2968
Cry11Aa1	M31737	Donovan et al., 1988	J Bact 170 4732-4738	41-1969
Cry11Aa2	M22860	Adams et al., 1989	J Bact 171 521-530	<1-235
Cry11Ba1	X86902	Delecluse, 1995	AEM 61 4230-4235	64-2238
Cry11Bb1	AF017416	Orduz et al., 1998	BBA 1388 267-272	97-2346
Cry12Aa1	L07027	Narva et al., 1991	EP 0462721	1->3771
Cry13Aa1	L07023	Narva et al., 1992	WO 92/19739	1-2409
Cry14Aa1	U13955	Narva et al., 1994	WO 94/16079	1-3558
Cry15Aa1	M76442	Brown & Whiteley, 1992	J Bact 174 549-557	1036-2055
Cry16Aa1	X94146	Barloy et al., 1996	J Bact 178 3099-3105	158-1996
Cry17Aa1	X99478	Barloy et al., 1998	Gene 211 293-299	12-1865
Cry18Aa1	X99049	Zhang et al., 1997	J Bact 179 4336-4341	1451-3571
Cry19Aa1	Y07603	Rosso & Delecluse, 1996	AEM 63 4449-4455	719-2662
Cry19Ba1	D88381	Hwang et al., 1998	SAB 21 179-184	626-2671
Cry20Aa1	U82518	Lee & Gill, 1997	AEM 63 4664-4670	60-2318
Cry21Aa1	I32932	Payne et al., 1996	USP 5589382	1-3501
Cry21Aa2	I66477	Feitelson, 1997	USP 5670365	1-3501
Cry22Aa1	I34547	Payne et al., 1997	USP 5596071	1-2169
Cry23Aa1	AF03048	Donovan & Slaney, 1998	WO 98/13498	

Table 2 (contd).

Name	Acc No	Reference	Journal	Coding
Cry24Aa1	U88188	Kawalek & Gill, 1998	Unpublished	1-2022
Cry25Aa1	U88189	Kawalek & Gill, 1998	Unpublished	1-2028
Cyt1Aa1	X03182	Waalwijk et al., 1985	NAR 13 8207-8217	140-886
Cyt1Aa2	X04338	Ward & Ellar, 1986	JMB 191 1-11	509-1255
Cyt1Aa3	Y00135	Earp & Ellar, 1987	NAR 15 3619-3619	36-782
Cyt1Aa4	M35968	Galjart et al., 1987	Curr Micro 16 171-177	67-816
Cyt1Ab1	X98793	Thiery et al., 1997	AEM 63 468-473	28-777
Cyt1Ba1	U37196	Payne et al., 1995	USP 5436002	1-795
Cyt2Aa1	Z14147	Koni & Ellar, 1993	JMB 229 319-327	270-1046
Cyt2Ba1	U52043	Guerchicoff et al., 1997	AEM 63 2716-2721	287-655
Cyt2Ba2	AF020789	Guerchicoff et al., 1997	AEM 63 2716-2721	<1->469
Cyt2Ba3	AF022884	Guerchicoff et al., 1997	AEM 63 2716-2721	<1->469
Cyt2Ba4	AF022885	Guerchicoff et al., 1997	AEM 63 2716-2721	<1->469
Cyt2Ba5	AF022886	Guerchicoff et al., 1997	AEM 63 2716-2721	<1->471
Cyt2Ba6	AF034926	Guerchicoff et al., 1997	AEM 63 2716-2721	<1->472
Cyt2Bb1	U82519	Cheong & Gill, 1997	AEM 63 3254-3260	416-1204

Most naturally occurring Bt strains contain ICPs active against a single order of insects. However, conjugative transfer between Bt strains or related species can occur, resulting in new strains with various plasmid contents. Thus the mobility of the *cry* genes and the exchange of plasmids may explain the diverse and complex activity spectra observed in Bt (González & Carlton, 1980; González et al., 1981; González et al., 1982; Reddy et al., 1987; Jarrett & Stephenson, 1990). New Bt strains have been developed by conjugation that are toxic to two insect orders.

2.1.6 Beta-exotoxin

Beta-exotoxin is associated with certain Bt subspecies (Btd, Btg, Btte and Btt), and products made from these Bt subspecies may contain the toxin (Cantwell et al., 1964; Mohd-Salleh et al., 1980). This heat-stable nucleotide, which is composed of adenine, glucose and allaric acid, inhibits RNA polymerase enzymes by acting competitively with ATP (Faust, 1973; Farkaš et al., 1977). Since RNA synthesis is a vital process in all life, beta-exotoxin exerts its toxicity for almost all forms of life tested including numerous insect species in the orders *Coleoptera*, *Diptera* and *Lepidoptera*. The presence of beta-exotoxin can be assayed using houseflies (*Musca domestica*) or high-performance liquid chromatography (HPLC) techniques (Campbell et al., 1987).

Table 3. Bt-associated toxins or toxin-like proteins that have not been assigned a name or entered into the nomenclature for the reasons given

Name	Accession	Journal	Coding region	Reason	Reference
Cry1i-like	I90732	USP 5723758	Peptide seq	Insufficient sequence data	Payne et al., 1998
Cry1-like	I90729	USP 5723758	Peptide seq	Insufficient sequence data	Payne et al., 1998
Cry9-like	AF093107	unpublished	<1->1917	Insufficient sequence data	Wasano & Ohba, 1998
40kda	M76442	J Bact 174 549-557	45-971	No reported toxicity	Brown & Whiteley, 1992
Cryc35	X92691	unpublished	1-981	No reported toxicity	Juarez-Perez et al., 1995
Crytdk	D86346	unpublished	177-2645	No reported toxicity	Hashimoto, 1996
Cryc53	X98616	unpublished	1-1005	No reported toxicity	Juarez-Perez et al., 1996
p21med	X98794	AEM 63 468-473	1-552	No reported toxicity	Thiery et al., 1997
ET34	AF038049	WO 98/13498		No reported toxicity	Donovan & Slaney, 1998
Vip3a(a)	L48811	PNAS 93 5389-5394	739-3105	Not a crystal protein	Estruch et al., 1996
Vip3a(b)	L48812	PNAS 93 5389-5394	118-2484	Not a crystal protein	Estruch et al., 1996

Table 4. *Bacillus thuringiensis* holotype toxins

Name	Old name	Name	Old name
Cry1Aa	CryIA(a)	Cry5Ac	
Cry1Ab	CryIA(b)	Cry5Ba	
Cry1Ac	CryIA(c)	Cry6Aa	CryVIA
Cry1Ad	CryIA(d)	Cry6Ba	CryVIB
Cry1Ae	CryIA(e)	Cry7Aa	CryIIIC
Cry1Af		Cry7Ab	CryIIICb
Cry1Ag		Cry8Aa	CryIIIE
Cry1Ba	CryIB	Cry8Ba	CryIIIG
Cry1Bb	ET5	Cry8Ca	CryIIIF
Cry1Bc	PEG5	Cry9Aa	CryIG
Cry1Bd	CryE1	Cry9Ba	CryIX
Cry1Be		Cry9Ca	CryIH
Cry1Ca	CryIC	Cry9Da	
Cry1Cb	CryIC(b)	Cry9Ea	
Cry1Da	CryID	Cry10Aa	CryIVC
Cry1Db	PrtB	Cry11Aa	CryIVD
Cry1Ea	CryIE	Cry11Ba	Jeg80
Cry1Eb	CryIE(b)	Cry11Bb	
Cry1Fa	CryIF	Cry12Aa	CryVB
Cry1Fb	PrtD	Cry13Aa	CryVC
Cry1Ga	PrtA	Cry14Aa	CryVD
Cry1Gb	CryH2	Cry15Aa	34kDa
Cry1Ha	PrtC	Cry16Aa	cbm71
Cry1Hb		Cry17Aa	cbm72
Cry1Ia	CryV	Cry18Aa	CryBP1
Cry1Ib	CryV	Cry19Aa	Jeg65
Cry1Ic		Cry19Ba	
Cry1Ja	ET4	Cry20Aa	
Cry1Jb	ET1	Cry21Aa	
Cry1Jc		Cry22Aa	
Cry1Ka		Cry23Aa	
Cry2Aa	CryIIA	Cry24Aa	Jeg72
Cry2Ab	CryIIB	Cry25Aa	Jeg74
Cry2Ac	CryIIC	Cry26Aa	
Cry3Aa	CryIIIA	Cry27Aa	
Cry3Ba	CryIIIB	Cry28Aa	
Cry3Bb	CryIIIBb	Cyt1Aa	CytA
Cry3Ca	CryIIID	Cyt1Ab	CytM
Cry4Aa	CryIVA	Cyt1Ba	
Cry4Ba	CryIVB	Cyt2Aa	CytB
Cry5Aa	CryVA(a)	Cyt2Ba	"CytB"
Cry5Ab	CryVA(b)	Cyt2Bb	

Bt containing beta-exotoxin is used for the control of houseflies in some countries, but regulatory agencies currently prohibit the use of beta-exotoxin for other purposes.

2.1.7 Other Bt metabolites

Commercial Bt products do not contain metabolites that are considered hazardous to humans and the environment. However, Bt, like other bacteria, may produce during the vegetative growth and sporulation stages an assortment of antibiotics, enzymes, metabolites and toxins that are biologically active and may have effects on both target and non-target organisms (NTOs).

Using a non-quantitative (Lund & Granum, 1997) commercial Bc enterotoxin immunoassay (Tecra), Damgaard (1995) reported that vegetative cells grown from spores of commercial Bt products excreted a diarrhoeal enterotoxin. Damgaard et al. (1996a) found by Vero cell assay that Bt isolated from food was enterotoxigenic. None of these investigations estimated the quantity or activity of enterotoxins produced by the Bt strains. However, Shinagawa (1990) investigated a number of Bc and Bt isolates with an immunological assay and concluded that 43% of the Bt isolates had the same level of enterotoxins as enterotoxic Bc. Tayabali & Seligy (1997) found that vegetative Bt obtained from commercial products caused extensive damage to cultivated insect cells.

At least three enterotoxic activities have been described in Bc (Agata et al., 1995; Lund & Granum, 1997), and some Bc isolates are known to produce an emetic toxin (Andersson et al., 1998). The emetic toxin is primarily associated with the Bc H-1 (Kramer & Gilbert, 1992; Nishikawa et al., 1996) serotype, and has not so far been associated with Bt isolates.

Alpha-toxin is a phospholipase C, which primarily affects the cell membrane phospholipids (Heimpel, 1954; Bonnefoi & Béguin, 1959). Gamma-toxin is toxic to sawflies (*Tenthredinidae*), but the mode of action of this heat-labile toxin has not been determined (Heimpel, 1967).

The so called "water-soluble toxin" paralyses *Lepidoptera* (Fast, 1971), and the "mouse factor exotoxin" is toxic to mice as well as to

Lepidoptera (Krieg, 1971). The modes of action of these toxins have not been delineated.

A novel Bt vegetative insecticidal protein (Vip3A) has been identified from the culture media of some Bt strains (Estruch et al., 1996).

Several Bt and Bc enzymes have been described which may play a role in non-target activity: phospholipase (Damgaard et al., 1996b), sphingomyelinase (Gilmore et al., 1989), protease (Hotha & Banik, 1997), chitinase (Sampson & Gooday, 1998), and haemolysin (Baida & Kuzmin, 1995).

2.2 Bioassays

2.2.1 *Spore counts*

Bacterial spore counts do not necessarily reflect the insecticidal activity of a Bt strain or Bt product because the number and amount of ICPs produced per bacterial cell can vary.

2.2.2 *International bioassay for ICPs*

The final formulation of each Bt product is bioassayed against an accepted international standard using a specific test insect (Dulmage et al., 1981; de Barjac & Larget-Thiery, 1984). Its potency is defined in ITU/mg product. The standardization allows comparison of different formulations in the laboratory. Currently, the larvicidal activity is expressed in terms of lethal doses (LD_{50}) or lethal concentrations (e.g., LC_{50}, LC_{90}) according to the bioassay method used. For example, when susceptible mosquito larvae are exposed to Bti ICP, they have an LC_{50} of approximately 10 ng/ml water. A Bti whole culture gives an LC_{50} of approximately 10^3 cells/ml for susceptible mosquito larvae while a 10^9 cells/ml culture does not affect any laboratory mammals exposed by various routes.

3. MODE OF ACTION ON TARGET INSECTS

3.1 Bioactivity of field isolates

The mode of action of Bt has been reviewed by Schnepf et al. (1998) and can be summarized in the following stages: 1) ingestion of sporulated Bt and ICP by an insect larva; 2) solubilization of the crystalline ICP in the midgut; 3) activation of the ICP by proteases; 4) binding of the activated ICP to specific receptors in the midgut cell membrane; 5) insertion of the toxin in the cell membrane and formation of pores and channels in the gut cell membrane, followed by destruction of the epithelial cells (Cooksey, 1971; Norris 1971; Fast, 1981; Huber & Lüthy, 1981; Lüthy & Ebersold, 1981; Smedley & Ellar, 1996); and 6) subsequent Bt spore germination and septicaemia may enhance mortality (Fig. 1).

The specific bioactivity of Bt is dominated by the ICPs that are encoded by the *cry* genes and are active against susceptible species in the insect orders *Coleoptera*, *Diptera* and *Lepidoptera*. Specific Bt activities against other insect orders (*Hymenoptera*, *Homoptera*, *Dictyoptera*, *Mallophaga*) and to nematodes (*Strongylida*, *Tylenchida*), mites (*Acari*), flatworms (*Digenea*) and protozoa (*Diplomonadida*) have been described (Feitelson, 1993; Zukowski, 1995). The ICP must be ingested to be effective against the target (Visser et al., 1993).

3.2 Mechanism of action of Bt formulations

The ICP-spore complexes of Bt are ingested by susceptible insect larvae. In the midgut the parasporal crystalline ICP is dissociated to the protoxin form, and the protoxin is then activated to a holotoxin by gut proteases (Warren et al., 1984; Jaquet et al., 1987; Aronson et al., 1991; Honée & Visser, 1993). Shortly afterwards, the gut becomes paralysed and the larva ceases to feed.

The ICP structure and function have been reviewed in detail by Schnepf et al. (1998). Binding of the ICP to putative receptors is a major determinant of ICP specificity and the formation of pores in the midgut epithelial cells is a major mechanism of toxicity (Van Frankenhuyzen, 1993).

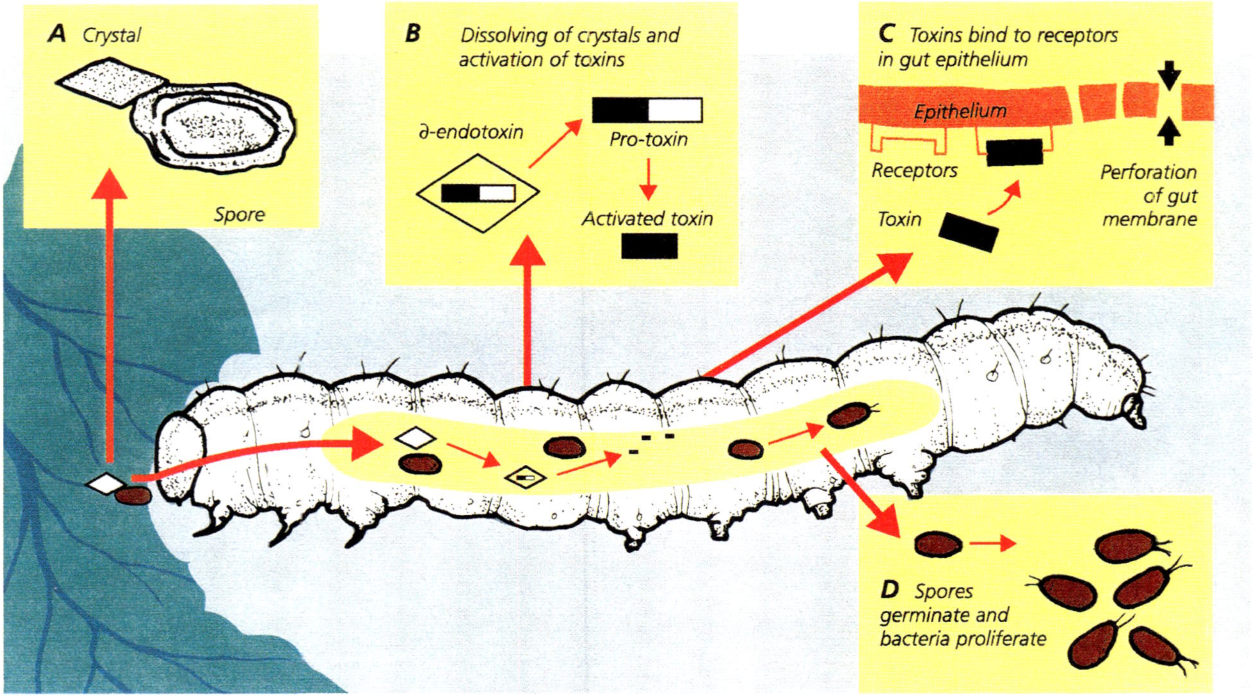

Fig 1. Mechanism of toxicity of Bt

The active toxin consists of three distinct domains (Höfte & Whiteley, 1989; Li et al., 1991; Grochulski et al., 1995). The three domains interact in a complex manner, but experimental data suggest that the C-terminal and middle domains of the toxin are involved in epithelial cell receptor binding and structural functions, while the N-terminal domain is primarily involved in ion channel and pore formation (Huber et al., 1981; Schnepf et al., 1998; Dean et al., 1996).

Binding to specific receptors has been demonstrated to be closely related to the insecticidal spectrum of the ICPs (Denolf et al., 1997). Van Rie et al. (1989) found the affinity of these toxins similar for the tobacco budworm (*Heliothis virescens*) and the tomato hornworm (*Manduca sexta*) brush border membrane vesicles, but the number of binding sites differed and reflected varied bioactivity. However, the toxin affinity for binding sites does not appear constant for all insects.

Pore or ion channel formation occurs after the binding to the receptor and insertion of the N-terminal domain into the membrane, whereby the regulation of the trans-membrane electric potential is disturbed. This can result in colloid-osmotic lysis of the cells, which is the main cytolytic mechanism that is common to all ICPs (Knowles & Ellar, 1987; Slatin et al., 1990; Schwartz et al., 1991; Schnepf et al., 1998). When the midgut epithelium of the larva is damaged, the haemolymph and gut contents can mix. This results in favourable conditions for the Bt spores to germinate. The resulting vegetative cells of Bt and the pre-existing microorganisms in the gut proliferate in the haemocoel causing septicaemia, and may thus contribute to the mortality of the insect larva.

3.3 Resistance of insect populations

A number of insect populations of several different species with different levels of resistance to Bt have been obtained by laboratory selection experiments during the last 15 years (Schnepf et al., 1998). The species include *Plodia interpunctella, Cadra cautella, Leptinotarsa decemlineata, Chrysomela scripta, Tricholplusia ni, Spodoptera littoralis, Spodoptera exigua, Heliothis virescens, Ostrinia nubilalis* and *Culex quinquefasciatus* (Schnepf et al., 1998) and resistance is shown to either Btk, Bti, Btte or other Bt subspecies.

During the last few years populations of the diamondback moth, *Plutella xylostella,* resistant to Btk and Bta have been found in heavily treated areas in numerous geographically isolated regions in the world, including Hawaii, Phillippines, Indonesia, Malaysia, Central America and some USA states (Schnepf et al., 1998). It is clear that this widespread appearance of resistance to Bt presents a cautionary tale for the way of using Bt and Bt toxin genes in pest management. Schnepf et al. (1998) have reviewed resistance management of Bt.

4. NATURAL AND TREATED HABITATS

The Bt subspecies represents a group of organisms that occur naturally and can be added to an ecosystem to achieve insect control (Andrews et al., 1987; Stahly et al., 1991). In this monograph, a natural habitat is considered to be one where Bt can be isolated when there has been no previous history of application of the organism to that ecosystem, whereas a treated habitat is one where Bt can be isolated after a previous history of application of the organism for insect control.

Insecticides formulated with Bt are being manufactured and used worldwide. These commercial Bt products may be applied as an insecticide to foliage, soil, water environments and food storage facilities. After application of Bt to an ecosystem, the organism may persist as a component of the natural microflora.

4.1 Natural occurrence of Bt

Members of the *Bacillus cereus* group can be found in most ecological niches. Hansen et al. (1996) reviewed the occurrence of Bt in the environment. Although the early Bt isolates were pathogenic for insects, it is now apparent that several Bt isolates have no known target (Ohba & Aizawa, 1986; Ohba et al., 1988; Hansen et al., 1996, 1998; Damgaard et al., 1997b). This lack of insecticidal activity may be attributed to the loss of ability to produce ICPs (Gordon, 1977), which may be due to a mutation in the ICP gene that could prevent expression (Klier & Lecadet, 1976; Stahly et al., 1978; Dean, 1984) or to the loss of ICP encoding sequences. Finally, the lack of known activity of a Bt crystalline toxin might simply be explained by a failure to test against the actual target organism. The list of Bt targets is still increasing. Although our knowledge of the activity of Bt populations in the environment is limited, a certain level of turn-over and vegetative growth must occur, as annual and seasonal variations in numbers and subspecies diversity of Bt populations have been observed (Damgaard et al., 1997b; Kim et al., 1998).

4.1.1 *Bt in insect hosts*

Numerous Bt subspecies have been isolated from dead or dying insect larvae and in most cases the isolate has toxic activity to the insect from which it was isolated (Goldberg & Margalit, 1977; de Barjac, 1981b; Hansen et al., 1996). These organisms have a narrow host range in the orders *Coleoptera*, *Diptera* and *Lepidoptera* and can proliferate within the bodies of their host insects. When the infected insect larva dies, the dead insect carcass usually contains relatively large quantities of spores and crystals that may be released into the environment (Prasertphon et al., 1973; Grassi & Deseö, 1984; Aly, 1985; Aly et al., 1985). Growth of Bt in non-target organisms has also been described. Eilenberg et al. (in press) found that Bt multiplication had occurred in non-target insects, which were also infected by insect pathogenic fungi.

Akiba (1986) reported recycling of naturally occurring Bt in insect cadavers when competitive microorganisms were at a low density. Outbreaks of Bt in susceptible insect populations occur relatively infrequently; most outbreaks have been limited to situations where the insect density is relatively high, providing better opportunity for establishing the disease within the insect population (Lynch et al., 1976; Burges & Hurst, 1977; Vaòková & Purrini, 1979; Margalit & Dean, 1985).

4.1.2 Bt in soil

The spores of Bt persist in soil, and vegetative growth occurs when nutrients are available (DeLucca et al., 1981; Akiba, 1986; Ohba & Aizawa, 1986; Travers et al., 1987; Martin & Travers, 1989).

DeLucca et al. (1981) found that Bt represented between 0.5% and 0.005% of all *Bacillus* species isolated from soil samples in the USA. Martin & Travers (1989) recovered Bt from soils globally. Meadows (1993) isolated Bt from 785 of 1115 soil samples, and the percentage of samples that contained Bt ranged from 56% in New Zealand to 94% in samples from Asia and central and southern Africa. Ohba & Aizawa (1986) isolated Bt from 136 out of 189 soil samples in Japan.

4.1.3 Bt on plant surfaces

Bt has been found extensively in the phylloplane. Numerous Bt subspecies have been recovered from coniferous trees, deciduous trees and vegetables, as well as from other herbs (Smith & Couche, 1991; Damgaard et al., 1997b). The Bt isolates have demonstrated a broad diversity both with specific activities to insects from the orders *Coleoptera* and *Lepidoptera* and with unknown activities (Smith & Couche, 1991; Damgaard et al., 1997b; Hansen et al., 1998). The bacterium has also been isolated from stored grain products (Meadows et al., 1992).

4.2 Treated habitats

Treated habitats are the locations where Bt insecticides (usually a mixture of spores and crystals) have been applied.

In Canada, Meadows (1993) estimated that approximately 10^{15} viable Btk spores per ha were released in a typical spray operation to control spruce budworm (*Choristoneura fumiferana)*.

4.3 Environmental fate, distribution and movement

Bt, like other members of the genus *Bacillus*, has the ability to form endospores that are resistant to inactivation by heat and desiccation and that persist in the environment under adverse conditions (Stahly et al., 1991). When considering the degradation of Bt in the environment, it is important to distinguish between changes in the numbers of viable spores and changes in biocidal activity. The survival and activity in the environment has been reviewed by Hansen et al. (1996).

The distribution and environmental transport of applied Bt formulations are influenced by the type of application and various environmental factors (Bulla et al., 1985; Andrews et al., 1987). Bt formulations are used in agriculture and forestry against coleopteran and lepidopteran pests and are usually directed towards the surface of plants, while the Bt formulations for control of dipteran pests (mosquitos and blackflies) are applied to their aquatic, larval habitats. Many Bt insecticides exhibit poor stability under field conditions, and so frequent reapplication is required (Griego & Spence, 1978; Sorenson & Falcon, 1980; Beegle et al., 1981).

4.3.1 Distribution and fate of Bt in terrestrial habitats

4.3.1.1 Fate of Bt and ICP on plant surfaces

Solar radiation appears to be the environmental factor most damaging to the stability of Bt ICP (Pinnock et al., 1974; Pinnock et al., 1977; Griego & Spence, 1978; Pusztai et al., 1991).

Griego & Spence (1978) demonstrated that Bt spores are inactivated rapidly when exposed to UV radiation, while Pusztai et al. (1991) demonstrated that the tryptophan residues of the Bt protoxin are damaged by solar radiation in the 300–380 nm range.

The combined effect of sunlight, leaf temperature and vapour pressure deficit appeared to contribute more to the reduction of bioactivity than any other single factor (Leong et al., 1980). Residue bioactivity may be detected up to 2 weeks after treatment with formulations containing UV protectants (Hostetter et al., 1975). Other studies on the effect of environmental exposure to Bt spores revealed that spore survival can be affected by the surface to which the material is applied.

Pinnock et al. (1974) reported that the half-life of Bt spores on leaves of California live oak (*Quercus agrifolia*) was 3.9 days, as compared to a half-life of 0.63 days when applied to leaves of western redbud (*Cercis occidentalis*).

Ignoffo (1992) summarized data for the reduction of spore viability and ICP activity on leaves of various plants in sunlight: Bt spore viability was reduced 80% in one day on red cedar leaves and 8% on soy bean leaves, while the ICP activity declined by 20% on red cedar leaves but 65% on soy bean leaves.

Dent (1993) reported that Bt formulations on foliage frequently have half-lives of up to 10 days. However, unformulated Bt may have a half-life of only a few hours. Pedersen et al. (1995) found that the initial spore half-life was 16 h during the first week after spraying cabbage with unformulated Btk.

There is also evidence that plant chemicals can inactivate Bt or influence infectivity. Lüthy (1986) demonstrated that extracts prepared from cotton leaves could inactivate ICPs.

Commercially applied Bt may persist at low levels for considerable periods of time. Reardon & Haissig (1983) reported that Btk was still present on balsam fir (*Abies balsamea*) one year after applications to control spruce budworm. The proliferation of spores through infection of susceptible insects should not be discounted as a source of low levels of Bt in treated areas. Several studies have demonstrated that Bt is able to grow and sporulate in insect cadavers (Meadows, 1993). From dead Egyptian cotton leafworm (*Spodoptera littoralis*), Jarrett & Stephenson (1990) isolated between 5.0×10^5 and 9.2×10^7 spores per larva.

Bt may be lost to the soil by overspray during application or by the action of rain on plant surfaces. Further losses arise from *in situ* degradation by environmental factors, such as ultraviolet (UV) radiation and microbial activity (Griego & Spence, 1978; Sorenson & Falcon, 1980; Beegle et al., 1981; West et al., 1984a,b). Pedersen et al. (1995) found that Bt was dispersed by rain splash from the soil to the lower leaves of cabbage.

4.3.1.2 *Fate of Bt in soil*

Petras & Casida (1985) reported that Bt spore counts in soil declined by a factor of ten in the first 2 weeks after application and then remained constant for 8 months. The response was similar in spores from commercial and laboratory cultures. In contrast, vegetative cells introduced into the soil persisted for only a short time. Soil pH had little effect on their survival. Spore persistence for more than 2 weeks apparently resulted from the inability of the spores to germinate in the soil.

Pedersen et al. (1995) sprayed unformulated Btk (1.2 5 10^4 cfu per g soil, spontaneous rifampicin-resistant mutant) on soil in 1993, and 2.3×10^3 cfu per g soil remained after 336 days. The field was left undisturbed, and 5½ years later spots with 1.5×10^3 Btk per g soil were found (Hansen & Hendriksen, 1999), but spots with very low Btk numbers were also recorded. These data indicate that the Btk had multiplied.

West et al. (1984a,b) reported that vegetative cells in soil disappeared at a rapid, exponential rate, whereas parasporal crystals disappeared at a slower, non-exponential rate, and spore numbers remained unaltered through 91 days of incubation at 25 °C, with no detectable germination. The proteinaceous crystalline protoxin of Bt has been shown to be degraded by soil microorganisms at an exponential rate with a half-life of about 3–6 days.

Saleh et al. (1970) reported that Bt spores could remain viable for several months in the soil and germinate when soil conditions favoured bacterial growth.

Bt spores do not appear to germinate readily in most soils and the crystalline protoxins are metabolized by other microorganisms. West et al. (1984a) reported that Bta in soil showed an exponential loss of insecticidal activity. The rate of loss was greater in non-sterile soil than in autoclaved soil. There was an initial rapid decrease, which stabilized at approximately 10% of the original inoculum level after 250 days incubation, until the cessation of sampling after two years. No loss of insecticidal activity was observed in autoclaved soil, which suggests that soil microorganisms were responsible for the loss of insecticidal activity in the natural, non-sterilized soil.

Several studies determined that Bt did not grow under most natural soil conditions (West et al., 1984a,b; Akiba, 1986). The data suggested that this was attributable to a failure of Bt spores to germinate in soil under these conditions. The spore is the only state in which Bt persists in natural soils.

An environmental fate study demonstrated no significant spore accumulation in either the organic or the mineral layers of soil over an 11-month period when Bt was applied aerially at 100 times the concentration used for operational programmes (Bernier et al., 1990).

Studies have indicated that Bt is relatively immobile in soil. Martin & Reichelderfer (1989) found no vertical movement beyond a 6-cm deep zone in soil and less than 10 m lateral movement, even along drainage courses.

Akiba (1991) reported a one-month irrigation study simulating the summer rainy season in Japan. There was no translocation of Bt below a depth of 10 cm. In soils receiving 45 cm simulated rainfall, Bt was detected to a depth of 3–6 cm. In tests using soil columns, Bt did not pass through a column of volcanic ash soil but a few spores were detected in flow-through water from an alluvial sand column. Results suggested that the major factor causing a decrease in the level of Bt was not a physical dilution due to the rainwater, but possibly an affinity of the spores for the soil particles.

Venkateswerlu & Stotsky (1992) reported that adsorption and binding of Bt toxin proteins to soil particles were greater on montmorillonite than on kaolinite clays. Maximum adsorption occurred within 30 min, and adsorption was not significantly affected by temperature between 7 °C and 50 °C.

4.3.2 *Distribution and fate of Bt in aquatic habitats*

Bti is often applied directly to water for the control of mosquitos and blackflies. Rapid sedimentation in all but the fastest flowing streams is regarded as an important limitation on the efficacy of such applications.

Sheeran & Fisher (1992) demonstrated that the sedimentation of Bti is facilitated by adsorption onto particulate material.

Ohana et al. (1987) found that spores may persist for at least 22 days in sediments, and the spores may be mobilized with such sediments during floods.

Btk has been reported to survive in fresh water and in seawater for more than 70 and 40 days, respectively, at 20 °C (Menon & De Mestral, 1985). A higher percentage of Btk was found to survive for extended periods in lake water than in tap and distilled water, presumably due to the presence of more nutrients in lake water. Bt has not been isolated from any drinking-water supplies.

Spores of Bti remained viable for shorter periods when suspended in moving water than when in static bottles, indicating that static laboratory trials may overestimate the longevity of these spores in the environment (Yousten et al., 1992).

Carcases of mosquito larvae killed by Bti have been shown to allow for the complete growth cycle (germination, vegetative growth and sporulation), thus becoming toxic themselves to scavenging yellow fever mosquito (*Aedes aegypti*) larvae (Khawaled et al., 1990).

Contact of Bti with mud can result in an immediate disappearance of larvicidal activity, but it has little influence on spore viability (Ohana et al., 1987). The cessation of toxicity was found to be caused by bacterial adsorption to soil particles, but the inactivation could be reversed by washing the mud away.

Special Bti formulations have been developed to prolong residence time of Bt at the surface or in the water column, where target insects feed.

Manasherob et al. (1998) found germination, growth and sporulation of Bti in excreted food vacuoles of a protozoan.

4.3.3 Transport of Bt by non-target organisms

In a field trial where Btk was sprayed on cabbage and soil, Pedersen et al. (1995) found that the Btk could be transported by non-target insects. Up to 10^3 cfu per g were found on surface-active insects, and carabid beetles carrying Btk were found up to 135 m from the Btk-treated area.

In a study of interactions between Bti and fathead minnows (*Pimephales promelas*), ingestion of Bt resulted in a high number of recoverable spores in the gastrointestinal tract and faeces (Snarski, 1990). Bti spore counts decreased rapidly after test fish were transferred to clean water, but spores were detected in low numbers in faeces for over 2 weeks. The data indicated that minnows could disperse Bt spores in the freshwater environment.

Meadows (1993) reported that, after the application of Bt on land, it may be dispersed by birds and mammals feeding on infected target insects. Some Bt-infected insect larvae may contain 6.6×10^8 to 4.2×10^9 spores per gram dry mass (Burges & Hurst 1977).

5. COMMERCIAL PRODUCTION

5.1 History of Bt and its commercial applications

5.1.1 *Production levels*

Conventional Bt products, which utilize naturally occurring or modified Bt strains, account for approximately 90% of the world MPCA market (Bernhard & Utz, 1993). Current annual production of Bt has been estimated at 3000 or more tonnes in developed countries. In China, up to 10 000 tons are produced annually (personal communication by Guan Xiong, Fujian Agricultural, University, 1997).

5.1.2 *Production processes, formulations and quality standards*

Bt products are produced using fermentation technology (Bernhard & Utz, 1993). Most commercial products contain ICP and viable Bt spores, but the spores are inactivated in some Bti products. During commercial-scale production of Bt products, there is little loss of bioactive components to the environment. The type of loss incurred is a function of the recovery method involved. No significant amount of bioactive component is lost from fermenter harvests if filtration is used to separate the insoluble solids (active ingredients) from the soluble liquid (inert) fraction of the harvest liquor, as shown by complete lack of bioactivity in the resulting liquid fraction. The liquid waste fractions may contain a low concentration of insoluble active component, but this is typically inactivated by processing in on-site waste treatment facilities. Although it is not a physical loss, measurable bioactivity is diminished if the recovered active material is processed through a dryer, due to the exposure of the bioactive components to the high temperatures required for drying. Guidelines for the handling of microorganisms during manufacture have been reviewed by Frommer et al. (1989).

Commercial Bt formulations include wettable powders, suspension concentrates, water dispersible granules, oil miscible suspensions, capsule suspensions and granules (Tomlin, 1997).

Quality standards for Bt fermentation products have been accepted by IUPAC (Quinlan, 1990). These standards include limits on the concentration of microbial contaminants and metabolites (Table 5).

Table 5. Maximum allowable levels of microbial contamination in bacterial insecticides (IUPAC Recommendation; Quinlan, 1990)

Types of microorganisms	Maximum concentrations
Viable mesophiles	<1 × 10^5/g
Viable yeasts and moulds	<100/g
Coliforms	<10/g
Staphylococcus aureus	<1/g
Salmonella	<1/10g
Lancefield Group D *Streptococci*	<1 × 10^4/g

In most cases strains of Bt that produce beta-exotoxins are not approved for commercial application, although some commercial use has been approved for control of certain fly species that are not susceptible to ICPs (Carlberg et al., 1985).

5.1.3 General patterns of use

Commercial applications of Bt have been directed mainly against lepidopteran pests of agricultural and forest crops; however, in recent years strains active against coleopteran pests have also been marketed (Table 6).

Strains of Bti active against dipteran vectors of parasitic disease organisms have been used in public health programmes.

5.1.3.1 *Applications in agriculture and forestry*

Commercial use of Bt on agricultural and forest crops dates back nearly 30 years, when it became available in France. Use of Bt has increased greatly in recent years and the number of companies with a commercial interest in Bt products has increased from four in 1980 to at least 18 (Van Frankenhuyzen, 1993). Several commercial Bt products with Bta, Btk or Btte have been applied to crops using conventional spraying technology (Table 6). Various formulations have been used on major crops such as cotton, maize, soybeans,

Table 6. Examples of commercial Bt products used against agricultural, forestry and public health pests
(Tomlin, 1997; see also the Internet site http://www.sipweb.org/bacteria.htm)

Bt sub-species	Commercial products	Producer
Bt (not defined)	Rijin	Scientific & Technological Development
Bt (not defined)	Bitayon	Jewin-Joffe Industry Ltd
Bt (not defined)	Delfin, Thuricide	SDS Biotech KK
Btk	Bactospeine, Biobit, Dipel, Foray	Abbott (USA)
	Bollgard	Ecogen/Crop Care
	Bactucide	Caffaro
	Baturad	Cequisa
	Condor, Crymax, Cutlass, Foil, Jackpot, Lepinox, Rapax, Raven	Ecogen
	Jackpot, Lepinox, Rapax	Intrachem
	Cordalene	Agrichem
	Larvo	Troy
	Costar, Delfin, Design, Javelin, Steward, Thuricide, Vault	Novartis/Thermo Trilogy Co
	Ecotech Bio, Ecotech Pro	Ecogen/Roussel-Uclaf
	Halt	Wockhardt
Bta	Xentari, Florbac	Abbott
	Certan	Novartis
Btte	Novodor	Abbott
Bti	Bactimos, Gnatrol, Vectobac	Abbott
	Acrobe	Cyanamid
	JieJueLing, MieJueLing	Huazhong Agricultural University
	Teknar	Novartis/ThermoTrilogy Co
Bt Ybt-1520	Mianfeng pesticide	Huazhong Agricultural University
Bt chinesensis	Shuangdo preparation	Huazhong Agricultural University
Btg	Spicturin	Tuticorin Alkali Chemicals and Fertilisers Ltd

potatoes, tomatoes, various crop trees and stored grains. Formulations have ranged from ultralow-volume oil to high-volume, wettable powder and aqueous suspensions. In the main, naturally occurring Bt strains have been used, but transgenic microorganisms expressing Bt toxins have been developed by conjugation and by genetic manipulation, and in some cases, these have reached the commercial market. These modified organisms have been developed in order to increase host range, prolong field activity or improve delivery of toxins to target organisms. For example, the coleopteran-active *cry*IIIA gene has been transferred to a lepidopteran-active Btk (Carlton et al., 1990). A plasmid bearing an ICP gene has been transferred from Bt to a non-pathogenic leaf-colonizing isolate of *Pseudomonas fluorescens*; fixation of the transgenic cells produces ICP contained within a membrane which prolongs persistence (Gelernter, 1990). The gene expressing *cry*IA(c) ICP has been inserted in *Clavibacter xyli* subspecies *cynodontis*, a bacterium that colonizes plant vascular systems. This has been shown to deliver the ICP effectively to European corn borer (*Ostrinia nubilalis*) feeding within plant stems (Beach, 1990). Improvements in performance arising from such modifications are such that transgenic organisms and their products are likely to be used much more widely in the future.

5.1.3.2 *Applications in vector control*

Bti has been used to control both mosquitos and blackflies in large-scale programmes (Lacey et al., 1982; Chilcott et al., 1983; Car, 1984; Car & de Moor, 1984; Cibulsky & Fusco, 1987; Becker & Margalit, 1993; Bernhard & Utz, 1993). For example, in Germany 23 tonnes of Bti wettable powder and 19 000 litres of liquid concentrate were used to control mosquitos (*Anopheles* and *Culex* species) between 1981 and 1991 in the Upper Rhine Valley (Becker & Margalit, 1993). In China, approximately 10 tonnes of Bti have been used in recent years to control the malarial vector, *Anopheles sinensis*.

The Onchocerciasis Control Programme of West Africa used more than five million litres of Bti from 1982 to 1997 to control blackflies (*Simulium damnosum*), the vector of the onchocerciasis filarial worm (*Onchocerca volvulus*), on the Upper Volta River System. The Programme was initially based solely on the control of the vector, *Simulium damnosum sensu lato*, by spraying the insecticide at breeding sites on river systems, where larval stages develop. At the peak of larvicidal activities about 50 000 km of rivers were treated in an area of over one million km^2 . The purpose was to interrupt the transmission of the parasite *Onchocerca volvulus*. The interruption of the cycle is achieved by destroying larval stages through aerial application of insecticides to breeding sites. Insecticide application was undertaken weekly (Moulinier et al., 1995). In order to assess the environmental impact of such treatments a network of sampling stations throughout the programme area were established.

Formulations of Bti range from wettable powder and fluid concentrates applied via conventional spray equipment from ground and air to slow-release briquet and tablet formulations. Examples of commercial Bti products are listed in Table 6.

6. EFFECTS ON ANIMALS

6.1 Mammals

Microbial pest control agents (MPCA) can, in principle, cause harmful effects via toxicity, inflammation, or a combination of these effects. The presence of bacteria in a specimen derived from tissues does not necessarily mean infection. *Colonization* refers to the multiplication of MPCA either on the surface or within an animal/human organism without causing any tissue damage. *Persistence* refers to the ability to recover the inoculum of the MPCA over time. Persistence and transient disturbances of the normal microbial flora are to be expected after exposure of experimental animals to MPCA, since clearance of the inoculum is not instantaneous. Persistence may not be equated with infection (Siegel & Shadduck, 1990). *Infection* by a MPCA means that there is evidence of the establishment and proliferation of the MPCA in tissues, coupled with tissue damage. Evidence of multiplication includes a measurable increase in the total amount of MPCA, recovery of vegetative stages when spores were administered, and failure of the inoculum to clear. It cannot be determined solely on the basis of lesions since injection of foreign material can elicit an inflammatory process (Siegel et al., 1987).

A classification of MPCA toxicity and infectivity has been proposed, in which MPCA is classified as toxic if an oral dose $\leq 10^6$ cfu per mouse causes mortality or clinical or pathological changes (Burges, 1980). However, any classification is very difficult because of the complexicity of the issue when dealing with living organisms (Ignoffo, 1973; Shadduck, 1983).

Older reports do not discriminate between different strains of Bt but modern molecular techniques have proven that variability exists within strains with the same serotype (Helgason et al., 1998; Hansen & Hendriksen, 1997a,b).

Mammalian toxicity studies on Bt-containing pesticides demonstrate that the tested isolates are not toxic or pathogenic (McClintock et al., 1995), as they occur in the products. Toxicity studies submitted to the US Environmental Protection Agency to support registration of Bt subspecies, and reviewed by McClintock et al. (1995), failed to show any significant adverse effects on body weight gain, clinical observations or upon necropsy.

Infectivity/pathogenicity studies have shown that the intact rodent system responds as expected to eliminate Bt gradually from the body after oral, pulmonary or intravenous challenge. However, clearance of Bti and Btk is not instantaneous. An intact immune system is not a prerequisite for clearance of Bti and Btk.

6.1.1 *Oral exposure*

In studies conducted with a single oral dose of laboratory grown Bt and commercial Bt formulations, there was no mortality associated with ingestion of Bti or Btk in mice and rats (Fisher & Rosner, 1959; de Barjac et al., 1980; Shadduck, 1980; Siegel et al., 1987) (Table 7).

Additionally, in data summarized by McClintock et al. (1995), no toxicity or infectivity was observed following oral administration of various Bt subspecies at doses of up to 4.7×10^{11} cfu/kg in rats.

In a study involving repeated oral exposure of mice and rats for 21 days with laboratory grown Bti, there was no mortality associated with ingestion of Bti and normal weight gain was observed in all treated rodents (de Barjac et al., 1980) (Table 8).

Hadley et al. (1987) conducted a study in which sheep were repeatedly treated with two commercial Btk formulations for 60 days. The only clinical sign was loose stools in sheep exposed to one Btk formulation. There was also microscopic evidence of moderate to marked lymphoid hyperplasia of the Peyer's patches in the caecum and colon of two out of six sheep treated with one Btk formulation and in one out of six sheep treated with the other Btk formulation. The authors did not consider these findings clinically significant.

Other multiple dose studies with Bt were summarized by McClintock et al. (1995). In rats, no toxicity or infectivity was associated with dietary exposure to Bti (4 g/kg per day) for 3 months. Administration of 1.3×10^{9} Btk spores/kg per day to rats by oral gavage was not toxic or infectious. McClintock et al. (1995) also reported the results of a 2-year study in which a commercial Btk preparation was fed to rats at 8400 mg/kg per day in the diet. Despite this excessive dose, the only effect observed was a decrease in body weight of females during weeks 10–104 of the study.

Table 7. Acute toxicity (single oral exposure) of Bt in experimental animals

Subspecies tested	Material tested	Test animal	Dose[a]	Mortality[b]	Reference
Btk	Washed cells, 24-h culture[c]	Rat, female, Sprague-Dawley	1.4×10^7cfu	0/6	Shadduck, 1980
Btk	Commercial product	Rat[d]	2×10^{11}cfu	0/10	Fisher & Rosner, 1959
Bti	48-h culture[c]	Mouse, female, Swiss	1.7×10^8cfu	0/20	de Barjac et al., 1980
Bti	48-h culture[c]	Rat, female, Wistar	3.4×10^7cfu	0/10	de Barjac et al., 1980
Bti	Washed cells[c], 24-h culture	Rat, female, Sprague-Dawley	6.9×10^7cfu	0/6	Shadduck, 1980
Bti	Washed commercial product	Rat, female, Sprague-Dawley	4×10^7cfu	0/10	Siegel et al., 1987

[a] All doses given are per animal
[b] Number dead/number treated
[c] Laboratory grown culture
[d] Breed and sex unknown

Table 8. Repeated dose (oral exposure) toxicity of Bt in mice, rats and sheep

Subspecies tested	Material tested	Test animal	Dose	Exposure time	Mortality[a]	Reference
Btk	Commercial product	Sheep, male, Rambouillet/Merino	1×10^{12}cfu	5 months	0/6	Hadley et al., 1987
Btk	Commercial product	Sheep, male, Rambouillet/Merino	1×10^{12}cfu	5 months	0/6	Hadley et al., 1987
Bti	48-h culture[b]	Mouse, female, Swiss	4.7×10^{10}cfu	21 days	0/20	de Barjac et al., 1980
Bti	48-h culture[b]	Rat, female, Wistar	1.2×10^{11}cfu	21 days	0/10	de Barjac et al., 1980

[a] Number dead/number exposed
[b] Laboratory grown culture

6.1.2 *Inhalation exposure*

These tests primarily address the potential infectivity of a MPCA. Inhalation is a likely route by which humans and animals may be exposed to Bt during application.

De Barjac et al. (1980) exposed 10 female Swiss mice for 12 min to 2×10^8 Bti spores (48-h laboratory grown whole culture). The mice were monitored for clinical signs for 15 days, and then killed. The lungs were removed aseptically and cultured for bacteria, but no Bti was recovered.

Siegel et al. (1987) exposed 27 female Sprague-Dawley rats to 2×10^6 spores of a commercial Bti formulation for 30 min. Rats were serially killed over a 27-day period and the lungs were cultured. Recovery of Bti declined from 5.92×10^3 cfu/g lung tissue at 3 h after exposure to none detected at 7 days after exposure. No gross lung lesions were observed.

Fisher & Rosner (1959) exposed 10 mice to 3×10^{10} spores of a commercial Btk product 4 times in a 6-day period. The Btk-treated mice exhibited no clinical signs during the treatment period and no gross pathological changes at necropsy.

6.1.3 *Dermal exposure*

This test is similar to the dermal exposure tests used in chemical toxicology. Bt does not have any external contact toxicity due to its mode of action, as shown in the following studies.

De Barjac et al. (1980) applied 5.1×10^7 cfu Bti of a 48-h laboratory grown culture to the skin of 20 female Swiss mice. No mortality was observed and there was no evidence of skin inflammation.

Other studies, reviewed by McClintock et al. (1995), indicate that Bt was not toxic or pathogenic to rabbits following dermal exposure to various Bt subspecies at doses of up to 2500 mg/kg. In some cases, mild irritation was observed.

6.1.4 Dermal scarification exposure

This test evaluates both the potential toxicity and infectivity of a MPCA. In the case of Bt, toxicity is unlikely due to its mode of action. However, this test also evaluates the importance of intact skin in preventing infection by Bt.

Fisher & Rosner (1959) scarified the skin of 4 rabbits, then applied 2.2×10^6 cfu of a commercial Btk formulation. No skin inflammation or sign of infection was observed.

De Barjac et al. (1980) applied 3.3×10^{13} cfu of a commercial Bti formulation to the skin of 6 male New Zealand White rabbits. No skin inflammation or sign of infection was observed.

6.1.5 Subcutaneous inoculation

This route of exposure is considered a more challenging test of potential infectivity than oral or dermal exposure, because the barrier of the skin is breached. However, subcutaneous exposure may take place only if the skin is damaged by the spraying or is already otherwise damaged.

De Barjac et al. (1980) subcutaneously inoculated 20 female Swiss mice and 10 tricolour guinea-pigs, respectively, with 8.5×10^7 cfu and 1.7×10^8 cfu of a 48-h laboratory-grown Bti culture. There was no evidence of infection and no mortality was observed.

Siegel et al. (1987) subcutaneously inoculated 15 female BALB/c mice with 1×10^9 cfu of a commercial Bti formulation. Abscesses occurred at the injection site but these were attributed to the introduction of high concentrations of heat-stable foreign material, since they also occurred when autoclaved Bti was injected. There was no evidence of infection and no mortality was observed.

6.1.6 Ocular exposure

The primary purpose of this procedure is to test for the irritancy of a MPCA, although this test also evaluates potential infectivity as well. In these tests, Bt may persist for days in rabbit eyes because of the depth of the conjunctival sac coupled with limited tear production by rabbits.

De Barjac et al. (1980) inoculated the eyes of six male New Zealand White rabbits with 3.7×10^7 cfu of a 48-h laboratory-grown Bti culture. No conjunctivitis or ocular irritation was observed. Siegel & Shadduck (1990) inoculated 12 female New Zealand White rabbits with 5.4×10^6 cfu of a commercial Bti formulation. No ocular irritation or conjunctivitis was observed and no Bti was recovered by swabbing after one week.

In data reviewed by McClintock et al. (1995), only mild irritation was observed following ocular administration of certain Bt subspecies to rabbits.

Siegel et al. (1987) inoculated the eyes of 6 male New Zealand White rabbits with 50 mg of a dry powder-commercial Bti formulation for 9 days, and another 6 male New Zealand White rabbits were treated with 50 mg of a laboratory-grown Bti culture for 9 days. No ocular irritation or conjunctivitis was observed in the rabbits that received the commercial powder. The rabbits that received the laboratory culture experienced severe conjunctival congestion and discharge. This was not attributed to Bti but rather to the nature of the inoculum. The laboratory strain was a dry paste with hard clumps while the commercial formulation was a soft powder.

6.1.7 *Intraperitoneal exposure*

The administration of a MPCA by this route is considered a highly challenging route of exposure. Human and animal exposure to Bt by this route is very unlikely to occur during the course of normal application of Bt. This route evaluates the ability of Bt to cause infection or produce toxic metabolites in the peritoneal cavity. Some of the safety studies that utilized this route of exposure also evaluated the clearance of Bt over time (Table 9).

Additional studies employing mice have been conducted using this route of exposure, which evaluates the role played by an intact immune system in preventing infection by Bt. These studies were deemed necessary to assess the risk posed by Bt to humans undergoing

Table 9. Acute toxicity of Bt after intraperitoneal injection of guinea-pigs, mice and rats

Subspecies tested	Material tested	Test animal	Dose	Mortality[a]	Reference
Btk	Washed cell, 24-h culture[b]	Rat, female, Sprague-Dawley	1.4×10^9cfu	0/6	Shadduck, 1980
Btk	Commercial product	Mouse	3×10^9cfu	0/5	Fisher & Rosner, 1959
Bti	48-h culture[b]	Mouse, female, Swiss	6.8×10^7cfu	0/20	de Barjac et al., 1980
Bti	48-h culture[b]	Guinea-pig, female, tricolour	1.7×10^7cfu	0/10	de Barjac et al., 1980
Bti	Washed cell[b], 24-h culture	Rat, female, Sprague-Dawley	6.9×10^7cfu	0/6	Shadduck, 1980
Bti	Washed commercial product	Rats, male and female Sprague-Dawley	4×10^7cfu	1/20	Siegel et al., 1987

[a] Number dead/number treated
[b] Laboratory grown culture

immunosuppressive chemotherapy and the risk posed by Bt to humans infected with the human immunodeficiency viruses. Immune suppression in mice was accomplished either by use of corticosteroids, which inhibited helper T-cells and selectively damaged B-cell activity, or through the use of athymic mice, which lack the functional T lymphocyte component of their immune system.

6.1.7.1 *Immune-intact animals*

De Barjac et al. (1980) intraperitoneally injected 100 female Swiss mice with 3.4×10^7 cfu of a 48-h laboratory-grown Bti culture and killed groups of 10 mice daily (Table 9). Blood samples were taken by cardiac puncture and Bt was recovered until day 8. No mortality was observed.

Fisher & Rosner (1959) intraperitoneally injected 30 mice of unspecified sex and strain with a laboratory-grown Btk culture and withdrew cardiac blood samples 24, 48 and 72 h after injection. There was no mortality and Btk was recovered as late as 48 h after injection from heart blood.

Siegel & Shadduck (1990) conducted three clearance studies using female CD-1 mice. In one experiment, 33 females were injected with 2.7×10^7 cfu of a washed commercial Bti formulation and serially killed over 80 days. Bti did not clear and was recovered from the heart blood on days 67 and 80. The investigators noted that the initial inoculum was composed of approximately 95% vegetative cells and that vegetative cells take longer to clear than spores. This was confirmed in a follow-up experiment in which two groups of 16 females each were injected with inocula containing 1.5×10^7 cfu of spores only or a 25% vegetative cell and 75% spore mixture. Both inocula cleared exponentially from the spleens of the mice but the 100% spore inoculum cleared sooner than did the inoculum that contained vegetative cells. These experiments demonstrated that Bti and Btk persist for a variable length of time in mice following injection but that they are cleared over time. These studies also suggest that the nature of the inoculum may play a role in the speed by which it is cleared.

Data summarized by McClintock et al. (1995) indicate that toxicity (100% mortality in extreme cases) may be observed following injection of ≥ 10^8 cfu of certain Bt subspecies intraperitoneally in mice. Lower doses (≤ 10^7 cfu/mouse) were non-toxic. Death generally occurred shortly after injection, indicating that an infectious process had not occurred. Although the basis for the toxicity observed at doses ≥ 10^8 cfu is not understood, these findings are not considered as evidence of a hazard associated with Bt products, since the route of administration is not relevant to human and animal exposure conditions.

6.1.7.2 *Immune-suppressed animals*

Siegel et al. (1987) injected 42 female BALB/c mice with 1.25 mg of a cortisone acetate twice weekly in order to suppress their immune system and subsequently injected them with 3.4×10^7 cfu of a washed commercial Bti formulation. Three cortisone-treated mice but none of the non-cortisone-treated mice died but this mortality was attributed to injury caused by injection. In the remaining 39 mice Bti was still recovered in the spleen 49 days after injection. In a companion experiment, 42 athymic mice were injected with the same dose of a washed commercial Bti formulation. Twenty-six of the 42 died within 5 to 10 h after injection; autopsy did not reveal the cause of death. In the surviving mice, Bti was recovered in the spleen 49 days after the injection. In a follow-up experiment, 30 athymic mice were injected with 2.6×10^7 cfu of another (washed) commercial Bti formulation and serially killed over a 36-day period. No mortality occurred. Bti was still recovered on day 36 after injection.

Siegel & Shadduck (1990) injected 24 athymic mice with 2.7×10^7 cfu of a washed commercial Bti formulation and evaluated clearance over a 27-day period. No mortality was observed and clearance was faster in the euthymic than athymic mice. Bti was still recovered 27 days after injection.

These experiments demonstrated that an intact immune system is not essential to prevent infection by Bti and Btk, but the kinetics of clearance differ between athymic and euthymic mice as well as between corticosteroid-treated and untreated euthymic mice. Based on these data, immune-suppressed individuals do not face any increased risk of infection by Bt.

6.1.8 Effects of activated Bt ICP

It has been demonstrated that the alkali-solubilized ICP from Bti is lethal when injected into mice (Thomas & Ellar, 1983). Alkali-solubilized Bti ICP was also cytolytic to human erythrocytes, mouse fibroblasts, and primary pig lymphocytes *in vitro* (Thomas & Ellar, 1983; Gill et al., 1987). This activity is attributed to a cytolytic factor encoded by *Cyt A* gene of Bti. Most other Bt subspecies lack this gene. Human exposure to activated Bti ICP is most unlikely.

6.1.9 Studies in wild animals

Numerous studies have been conducted on wild animals as part of the registration process. Most of the data are proprietary and not publicly available. No adverse effects have been reported.

In Canada, Innes & Bendell (1989) studied the effect of a commercial Btk formulation on small mammal populations in woodland. Populations of eight species of rodents (*Clethrionomys gapperi*, *Eutamius minimus*, *Microtus chrotorrhinus*, *Napaeozapus insignis*, *Peromyscus maniculatus*, *Phenacomys intermedius*, *Tamias striatus* and *Zapus hudsonius*) and four species of shrew (*Blarina brevicauda*, *Sorex cinereus*, *Sorex fumeus* and *Sorex hoyii*) were studied by trapping over a 3-month period and shown to be unaffected when compared to populations from untreated areas. This suggests that the ingestion of infected insects by shrews had no immediate effects on their populations.

6.2 Effects on birds

In a number of studies (Table 10), the acute toxicity and pathogenicity of commercial Bta, Bti, Btk and Btte formulations for young bobwhite quail (*Colinus virginianus*) and young mallards (*Anas platyrhynchus*), when administered daily by oral gavage at high dosages, were evaluated (Beavers et al., 1989a,b; Lattin et al., 1990a,b,c,d; Beavers, 1991a,b). The Bt-treated birds showed no apparent toxicity or pathogenicity. In those studies which also evaluated feed consumption and weight gain, the Bt-treated birds showed no effect when compared with the non-treated controls.

Table 10. Effects of oral 5-day exposure of Bt on birds

Materials tested[a]	Species	Dose	Results	Reference
Bta	*Colinus virginianus*	1714 mg (3.4 × 10^{11} cfu)/kg/day	no toxicity or pathogenicity observed	Beavers, 1991b
	Anas platyrhynchus	1714 mg (3.4 × 10^{11} cfu)/kg/day	no toxicity or pathogenicity observed	Beavers, 1991a
Bti	*Colinus virginianus*	3077 mg (3.4 × 10^{11} cfu)/kg/day	no toxicity or pathogenicity observed	Lattin et al., 1990d
	Anas platyrhynchus	3077 mg (6.2 × 10^{11} cfu)/kg/day	no toxicity or pathogenicity observed	Lattin et al., 1990b
Btk	*Colinus virginianus*	2857 mg (5.7 × 10^{10} cfu)/kg/day	no toxicity or pathogenicity observed	Lattin et al., 1990a
	Anas platyrhynchus	2857 mg (5.7 × 10^{10} cfu)/kg/day	no toxicity or pathogenicity observed	Lattin et al., 1990c
Btte	*Colinus virginianus*	740 mg (4 × 10^{9} spores)/kg/day	no toxicity or pathogenicity observed	Beavers et al., 1989a
	Anas platyrhynchus	740 mg (4 × 10^{9} spores)/kg/day	no toxicity or pathogenicity observed	Beavers et al., 1989b

[a] commercial preparation

In Canada, Buckner et al. (1974) assessed the impact of Btk on breeding bird populations (13–14 families, 33–34 species) during a field trial for spruce budworm control. The bird populations in 10-ha control and treated plots were measured before and daily for 3 weeks after application. No differences were detected between the populations in the control and treated plots.

In the USA, Gaddis & Corkran (1986) evaluated the effect of a Bt spray programme on the reproductive performance of the chestnut-backed chickadee (*Parus rufescens*). This study was undertaken to determine if secondary effects on the chickadces would result from the possible reduction of lepidopteran species, which contribute to the diet of this species. The data showed no treatment-related effect on the number of eggs per nest, percentage of eggs hatched, percentage of young fledged, percentage of nests fledging at least one young, or the body weight of the nestlings.

6.3 Effects on aquatic vertebrates

The World Health Organization (WHO, 1982) reviewed laboratory and field studies, performed by that time, that examined the impact of Bt on frogs (*Hyla regilla, Rana temporaria*), goldfish (*Carassius auratus*), mosquito fish (*Gambusia affinis*), newts (*Taricha torosa, Triturus vulgaris*), rainwater killifish (*Lucania parva*) and toads (*Bufo* species). No adverse effects were reported.

Under static renewal conditions, Boeri (1991) exposed rainbow trout (*Oncorhynchus mykiss*) to high concentrations (100 mg/litre) of a commercial Bta formulation for 96 h and observed no adverse effects (Table 11).

Under static renewal conditions, Surprenant (1989) exposed rainbow trout (*Oncorhynchus mykiss*) to high concentrations (100 mg/litre) of a commercial Btte formulation for 96 h and observed no adverse effects (Table 11).

During 30- or 32-day static renewal tests, bluegill sunfish (*Lepomis macrochirus*), sheepshead minnow (*Cyprinodon variegatus*) and rainbow trout (*Oncorhynchus mykiss*) were exposed to commercial Bti, Btk or Btte formulations at aqueous and dietary concentrations from 100 to 500 times the expected environmental concentrations

Table 11. Effects of Bt on fish

Material tested[a]	Species	Concentration	Duration	Results	Reference
Bta	*Oncorhynchus mykiss*	100 mg/litre water	96 h	No-observed-effect level	Boeri, 1991
Btk	*Lepomis macrochirus*	2.9×10^9cfu/litre water[b] 1.2×10^{10}cfu/g diet[c]	32 days	No significant toxicity or pathology	Christensen, 1990a
	Oncorhynchus mykiss	2.9×10^9cfu/litre water[b] 1.1×10^{10}cfu/g diet[c]	32 days	20% mortality but not infectivity	Christensen, 1990b
	Cyprinodon variegatus	2.6×10^{10}cfu/litre water[c] 3.3×10^9cfu/g diet[c]	30 days	No significant toxicity or pathology	Christensen, 1990c
Bti	*Lepomis macrochirus*	1.2×10^{10}cfu/litre water[c] 1.3×10^{10}cfu/g diet[c]	30 days	No significant toxicity or pathology	Christensen, 1990f
	Oncorhynchus mykiss	1.1×10^{10}cfu/litre water[c] 1.7×10^{10}cfu/g diet[c]	32 days	No significant toxicity or pathology	Christensen, 1990g
	Cyprinodon variegatus	1.3×10^{10}cfu/litre water[c] 2.1×10^{10}cfu/g diet[c]	30 days	No significant toxicity or pathology	Christensen, 1990h
Btte	*Salmo gairdneri*	100 mg/litre water	96 h	No-observed-effect level	Surprenant, 1989
	Oncorhynchus mykiss	1.6×10^{10} cfu/litre water[c] 1.34×10^{10}cfu/g diet[c]	30 days	No significant toxicity or pathology	Christensen, 1990d
	Cyprinodon variegatus	9.94×10^9cfu/g diet	30 days	No significant toxicity or pathology	Christensen, 1990e

[a] commercial formulations
[b] nominal concentration
[c] measured average concentration

(Table 11) (Christensen, 1990a,b,c,d,e,f,g,h). The results of these studies indicated that exposure to very high concentrations of Bti, Btk and Btte did not adversely affect the survival of these fish, nor did it produce lesions. In the Btk study, the rainbow trout had a 20% mortality during the last 4 days of the study (Christensen,1990b). This effect was attributed to the excessive competition for food that resulted from poor visibility due to the turbidity and the presence of suspended solids encountered in the water.

In Canada, Buckner et al. (1974) assessed the impact of Btk on brook trout (*Salvelinus fontinalis* Mitchell), common white suckers (*Catostomus commersoni* Lacepede) and smallmouth bass (*Micropterus dolomieui* Lacepede) during a field trial for spruce budworm control. The fish populations were assessed visually in underwater surveys before and after the spray programme. No effect on their populations was seen.

Two analyses of surveys of the impact of the larvicidal campaign in the Onchocerciasis Control Programme of West Africa, which compared fish populations during the programme with the normal yearly fluctuation, observed little or no effects on the non-target populations. However, few details were provided (Yameogo et al., 1988; Levêque et al., 1988; Calamari et al., 1998).

6.4. Effects on invertebrates

6.4.1 *Effects on invertebrates other than insects*

The World Health Organization (WHO, 1982), reviewed laboratory and field studies performed up to that time that examined the impact of Bt on aquatic invertebrates, which included bivalve mollusks (oyster larvae, *Crassostrea gigas, Ostrea edulis*), copepods, decapods, flatworms, isopods, gastropods and ostracods. Of these organisms, only a few demonstrated any adverse effects.

In Canada, Buckner et al. (1974) evaluated the impact of Btk on a number of aquatic invertebrates during a field trial for control of the spruce budworm. Populations of *Amphipoda* (amphipods), *Decapoda* (crayfish), *Hydracarina* (water-mites), *Hirudinea* (leeches), *Hydrozoa* (freshwater hydra), *Nematoda* (roundworms), *Oligochaeta* (segmented worms), *Porifera* (freshwater sponges), *Pulmonata* (freshwater snails) and *Turbellaria* (flatworms) were determined by sampling 14 days prior to and up to 28 days after treatment. The populations of these aquatic invertebrates were not affected by the Btk treatment.

Benz & Altwegg (1975) studied the impact of Bt treatment at 100 times the recommended rate on populations of the earthworm *Lumbricus terrestris* and found no effect.

Horsburgh & Cobb (1981) reported that populations of the two-spotted spider mite (*Tetranchus urticae*) and *Panonychus ulmi* were not affected by biweekly sprays with a commercial Btk product.

Weires & Smith (1977) determined that sprays of a commercial Btk product on apples during a 4-month season had no effect on the two-spotted spider mite (*Tetranchus urticae*) and *Panonychus ulmi,* or on two predatory mites (*Amblyseius fallacis* and *Zetzellia mali*).

6.4.2 Effects on non-target insects

An extensive literature exists on the consequences of exposure of NTOs to Bt, including reports of several long-term field studies. The data have been reviewed periodically (e.g., WHO, 1982; Lacey & Mulla, 1990; Melin & Cozzi, 1990; Molloy, 1992; Otvos & Vanderveen, 1993). The range of non-target species that have been found to be susceptible to direct toxic action of Bt has remained small. A list of non-target species found to be insensitive to Btte was issued by Keller & Langenbruch (1993). In more than 30 years of commercial use, no serious, direct effects on NTOs have been reported as arising from Bt-based MPCAs. Several studies which identified effects of Bt on predators or parasitoids of susceptible insect species are listed by Navon (1993), but the effects have been small. Mortality in bees has been observed after exposure to vegetatively growing Bt but the effect does not seem to be related to spores or ICPs.

6.4.2.1 *Aquatic insects*

Bti is specific in its toxicity to dipterans. Nevertheless, many studies have tested the effect of Bti applications on a wide range of aquatic insects.

Lacey & Mulla (1990) summarized a number of studies of the effects of Bti on certain non-target arthropod species and arthropod populations in the laboratory and field (Table 12). The results of representative studies are summarized below.

Table 12. Effects of Bti on non-target arthropods[a]

Arthropod order	Type of study	Result[a]	References
Coleoptera	Laboratory	–	Schnetter et al., 1981
	Field	–	Mulla et al., 1982; Mulligan & Schaefer, 1982; Mulla, 1988
Diptera (*Chironomidae*)	Laboratory	+	Garcia et al., 1980; Ali, 1981; Ali & Baggs, 1981; Schnetter et al., 1981
	Field	+	Mulla et al., 1971; Ali, 1981; Mulligan & Schaefer, 1982; Rogatin & Baizhanov, 1984
	Field	–	Miura et al., 1980
Ephemeroptera	Laboratory	–	Ali, 1980; Schnetter et al., 1981; Mulligan & Schaefer, 1982
	Field	–	Schnetter et al., 1981; Mulla et al., 1982, Mulligan & Schaefer, 1982; Mulla, 1988
Heteroptera (*Corixidae*)	Field	–	Schnetter et al., 1981; Mulligan & Schaefer, 1982
Heteroptera (*Notonectidae*)	Laboratory	–	Schnetter et al., 1981; Olejnicek & Maryskova, 1986; Aly & Mulla, 1987
	Field	–	Mulla et al., 1982; Mulligan & Schaefer, 1982; Mulla, 1988
	Field	+	Purcell, 1981
Odonata	Laboratory	–	Mulla & Khasawinah, 1969; Mulligan & Schaefer, 1982; Aly, 1985; Aly & Mulla, 1987
	Field	–	Mulla, 1988

[a] – = no effect reported; + = an effect was reported, but does not necessarily imply that either individual arthropods or populations of arthropods were adversely affected.

Four species of chironomid larvae (*Chironomus crassicaudatus*, *Chironomus decorus*, *Glyptotendipes paripes*, *Tanytarsus* species) were tested with four Bti preparations. The chironomid larvae were less susceptible to Bti, being 13- to 75-fold more tolerant than mosquito larvae to the various Bti preparations (Ali, 1981; Ali & Baggs 1981). Garcia et al. (1980) induced low to high levels of mortality in some nematocerous *Diptera*, including a variety of taxa in the families *Ceratopogonidae*, *Chironomidae* and *Dixidae*, using dosages of Bti that were 50 to several hundredfold higher than concentrations used for mosquito control. Schnetter et al. (1981) reported complete mortality in chironomid larvae (*Chironomus thummi*) exposed to high levels of Bti for 48 h without food. Field-collected adult aquatic beetles exposed to Bti suffered little or no mortality (Schnetter et al., 1981). Ali (1980) tested a Bti formulation at 20 times the larvicidal dosage for mosquitos and reported no adverse effects against larval mayflies (*Baetis* species). Schnetter et al. (1981) reported that mayflies (*Cloeon* species) suffered no mortality when fed Bti at high dosages.

Aly & Mulla (1987) fed Bti intoxicated mosquito larvae (*Culex quinquefasciatus*) to field-collected fourth to fifth instar back-swimmers (*Notonecta undulata*). The predators were fed at the rate of 10 larvae per predator per day for 4 days, then the predators were fed unintoxicated mosquito larvae and observed for 15 to 17 days. The nymph and adult notonectids exhibited no adverse effects. Olejnicek & Maryskova (1986) observed no marked mortality in backswimmers (*Notonecta glauca*) that were fed Bti intoxicated mosquito larvae. Schnetter et al. (1981) found no mortality in backswimmers (*Notonecta glauca*) exposed for 48 h to high levels of Bti.

Mosquito larvae intoxicated with extremely high dosages of Bti were fed to naiads of the dragonfly *Tarnetrum corruptum* and damselfly *Enallagma civile*; the duration of development of the dragonfly and damselfly naiads, from the time of exposure to emergence, was not affected (Aly, 1985; Aly & Mulla, 1987)

Merritt et al. (1989) reported no evident of effects on the drift of aquatic invertebrates, or on the numbers of these invertebrates in benthic Surber samples, during a blackfly (*Simulium* species) control programme. In the USA, Molloy (1992) reviewed ten field trials where Bti was used against blackfly (*Simulium* species) larvae. He concluded that, although there was a potential for adverse impact of Bti on filter-feeding chironomids, the impact on stream insect communities overall was very small.

Over a three-season period, Bti administered at mosquito larvicidal rates had no adverse effects on the larvae of diving beetles (*Dytiscidae*) or water scavengers (*Hydrophylidae*) (Mulla et al., 1982; Mulla, 1988).

The application of a Bti formulation in a wildlife marsh showed no adverse effects on beetle larvae (Mulligan & Schaefer, 1982).

Ali (1981) evaluated the efficacy of various levels of a Bti formulation against chironomids in the families Chironominae and Tanytarsinae and obtained mortality at dosages higher than those employed to control mosquito larvae. Miura et al. (1980), using mosquito larvicidal dosages of a commercial Bti product, showed no reduction in the field populations of chironomids following treatment. Mulla et al. (1971) reported marked reductions in some chironomid populations, using a commercial Bti product at rates of 20 to 40 times the mosquitocidal rates. Mulligan & Schaefer (1982) reported a 40 to 70% reduction in some chironomid species after application of a Bti formulation to a wildlife marsh. Rogatin & Baizhanov (1984) noted a significant reduction of chironomids after Bti exposure.

Extensive quantitative observations were made on mayfly nymphs, mostly *Callibaetis pacificus*, but no notable effects were observed when Bti was applied against mosquito larvae (Mulla et al., 1982; Mulla, 1988). Mulligan & Schaefer (1982) found that Bti did not adversely affect mayfly nymphs (*Callibaetis* species). Schnetter et al. (1981) reported that mayflies (*Cloeon* species) were not affected when Bti was used in floodwater mosquito (*Aedes vexans*) larval habitats. Schnetter et al. (1981) collected water boatmen (*Corisella* species) from mosquito larval habitats on the upper Rhine river in Germany. The water boatman population was not affected after exposure to Bti for 48 h. Adverse effects were noted on backswimmers (*Buenoa* species, *Notonecta undulata*, and *Notonecta unifasciata*) during field trials with Bti (Mulla et al., 1982; Mulla, 1988). Mulligan & Schaefer (1982) reported that the backswimmer (*Notonecta* species) populations in a wetland marsh were not adversely affected by the application of a Bti formulation. Purcell (1981) noted reductions in populations of backswimmers (*Buenoa elegans*, *Notonecta indica)* after application of Bti, but attributed this to the flying activity of these predators.

No adverse effects on naiads of the dragonfly (*Tarnetrum corruptum*) and damselfly (*Enallagma civile*) were reported when Bti was used against larval mosquito populations (Mulla & Khasawinah, 1969; Mulla, 1988).

No notable reduction in the number of nymphs of several species of dragonfly (*Anisoptera*) and damselfly (*Zygoptera*) occurred when Bti was applied in a wetland marsh (Mulligan & Schaefer, 1982).

In the follow-up to the Onchocerciasis Control Programme of West Africa (section 5.1.3.2), little or no effect on the non-target populations was observed. However, few details were provided (Yameogo et al., 1988; Levêque et al., 1988; Calamari et al., 1998).

6.4.2.2 *Terrestrial insects*

Melin & Cozzi (1990) summarized a number of studies on the effects of Btk, Btg, Btt and Bte on non-target arthropod species and arthropod populations in the laboratory and field. Representative studies on Btk, Btg, Btt and Bte are listed in Tables 13 and 14.

Obadofin & Finlayson (1977) determined that a commercial Btk product had a minimal effect on the ground beetle (*Bembidion lampros*). Wilkinson et al. (1975) evaluated the contact activity of a commercial Btk product for 5 days at levels equivalent to field rates on an adult ladybird beetle (*Hippodamia convergens*) and found no adverse effects.

Workman (1977) exposed earwigs (*Labidura riparia*) to a commercial Btk product at rates equivalent to 10 times the normal field application rate. No mortality was observed in these predators.

Hamed (1978–1979) found that two tachinid species (*Bessa fugax* and *Zenilla dolosa*) were not affected after being fed suspensions of a commercial Btk product. Horn (1983) observed a reduction in the number of syrphid larvae on collards sprayed with a commercial Btk

Table 13. Effects of Btk on non-target arthropods

Arthropod order	Type of study	Results[a]	References
Acarina	Field	–	Weires & Smith, 1977; Horsburgh & Cobb, 1981
Coleoptera	Laboratory	–	Wilkinson et al., 1975; Obadofin & Finlayson, 1977
	Field	–	Harding et al., 1972; Buckner et al., 1974; Johnson, 1974; Wallner & Surgeoner, 1974; Asquith, 1975
Dermaptera	Laboratory	–	Workman, 1977
Diptera	Laboratory	–	Hamed, 1978–1979
	Laboratory	–	Horn, 1983
	Field	–	Dunbar et al., 1972; Fusco, 1980
Heteroptera	Laboratory	–	Hamed, 1978–1979
	Field	–	Harding et al., 1972; Elsey, 1973; Jensen, 1974; Wallner & Surgeoner, 1974
Hymenoptera (Honey-bees)	Laboratory	–	Krieg, 1973
	Laboratory	–	Krieg et al., 1980
	Field	–	Buckner et al., 1974
Hymenoptera (Parasitoids)	Laboratory	–	Wallner & Surgeoner, 1974; Hassan & Krieg, 1975; Krieg et al., 1980
	Laboratory	+	Dunbar & Johnson, 1975; Mück et al., 1981; Weseloh & Andreadis, 1982; Wallner et al., 1983; Thomas & Watson, 1986
	Field	–	Dunbar et al., 1972; Buckner et al., 1974; Wanller & Surgeoner, 1974; Hamel, 1977; Morris et al., 1977; Morris et al., 1980; Fusco, 1980
	Field	+	Weseloh et al., 1983
Neuroptera	Laboratory	–	Wilkinson et al., 1975; Hassan, 1983
Dictyoptera (mantis)	Laboratory	–	Yousten, 1973

[a] – = no effect reported; + an effect was reported, but does not imply that either individual arthropods or populations of arthropods were adversely affected.

Table 14. Effects of different Bt strains on non-target arthropods

Arthropod order	Type of study	Result[a]	References
Btg			
Hymenoptera (Honey-bees)	Laboratory	–	Cantwell & Shieh, 1981
	Field	–	Burges, 1977
	Field	–	Burges & Bailey, 1968
Btt			
Coleoptera	Field	+	Kazakova & Dzhunusov, 1977
Hymenoptera (Honey-bees)	Laboratory	+	Krieg & Herfs, 1963; Krieg, 1973
	Laboratory	–	Martouret & Euverte, 1964; Cantwell et al., 1966
Hymenoptera (Parasitoids)	Laboratory	+	Hassan & Krieg, 1975; Salama et al., 1982; Hassan, 1983; Salama & Zaki, 1983
	Laboratory	–	Krieg et al., 1980
Bte			
Coleoptera	Laboratory	–	Salama & Zaki, 1983
	Laboratory	+	Salama et al., 1982
Hymenoptera (Parasitoids)	Laboratory	+	Salama & Zaki, 1983
Neuroptera	Laboratory	+	Salama et al., 1982

[a] – = no effect reported; + = an effect was reported, but does not imply that either individual arthropods or populations of arthropods were adversely affected.

product. This effect was attributed to a repellent effect on the syrphid adults.

Hamed (1978–1979) found that *Picromerus bidens* was not adversely affected after feeding upon lepidopteran larvae (*Yponomeuta evonymellus*) that had fed upon leaves treated with commercial Btk products.

Hassan (1983) determined a commercial Btk product to be harmless to adult lacewings (*Chrysopa carnea*) when they were exposed at normal field rate concentrations. Wilkinson et al. (1975) found negligible mortality in larval or adult lacewings (*Chrysopa carnea*) when a commercial Btk product was applied as a contact spray at recommended field rates.

Yousten (1973) fed lethal quantities of Btk to larval cabbage loopers (*Trichoplusia ni*) and just prior to death offered these larvae to young Chinese praying mantids (*Tenodera aridifolia* subspecies *sinensis*). The mantids were not susceptible to the spore-crystal mixtures in the intact insect host.

Asquith (1975) found that black ladybird beetles (*Stethorus punctum*) on apple trees were not affected by treatment with a commercial Btk product. Buckner et al. (1974) monitored populations of ground beetles following aerial spraying of spruce with two commercial Btk products and found no effect on these predators. Harding et al. (1972) detected no reduction in population levels of ladybird beetles (coccinellids), rove beetles (staphyllinids), or checkered beetles (clerids) in plots treated with a commercial Btk product. Johnson (1974) evaluated several commercial Btk products as both sprays and baits on tobacco. During the 2-year study, the populations of two coccinellids (*Hippodamia convergens* and *Colemegilla maculata*) were not affected by the microbial treatments. Wallner & Surgeoner (1974) found no effects on coccinellids (*Cycloneda munda*, *Chilocorus bivulnerus* and *Adalia bipuncta*) following forest sprays with a commercial Btk product.

While evaluating a commercial Btk product for the control of gypsy moth (*Lymantria dispar*) and elm spanworm (*Ennomos subsignacius*), Dunbar et al. (1972) found no adverse effect on two tachinids (*Blepharipa scutellata* and *Parasitigena agilis*). Fusco (1980) reported an increased incidence of parasitism by two tachinids (*Blepharipa pratensis* and *Compsilura concinnata*) when Btk was applied in a field study.

Elsey (1973) reported no detrimental effect on spined stiltbug nymphs or adults (*Jalysus spinosus*) during a 2-month field study with a commercial Btk product. Harding et al. (1972) conducted a 2 year study to evaluate the effects of Btk on the natural enemies of the bollworm (*Helicoverpa zea*) on cotton (*Gossypium hirsutum*). Following applications of Btk against this pest, they reported no detectable effects on *Anthocoridae* (minute pirate bugs, *Orius* species), *Lygaediae* (bigeyed bugs, *Geocoris* species), *Nabidae* (damsel bugs, *Nabis* species), or *Reduviidae* (assassin bugs). Jensen (1974) used a commercial Btk product on soybeans (*Glycine canescens*) to control the green cloverworm (*Plathypena scabra*) and the velvetbean caterpillar (*Anticarsis gemmitalis*). No adverse effect was observed on *Lygaediae* (bigeyed bugs, *Geocoris* species) or *Nabidae* (damsel bugs, *Nabis* species).

Wallner & Surgeoner (1974) found no effect on the spined soldier bug (*Podisus maculiventris*), following forest sprays of commercial Btk products to control the oakleaf caterpillar (*Heterocampa manteo*).

Although many data exist, in a review of the effects of the use of Btk in Canada, Addison (1993) concluded that few studies on NTOs had used soil invertebrate species and soil conditions relevant to field conditions in Canadian forests.

Salama & Zaki (1983) reared cotton leafworm larvae (*Spodoptera littoralis*) on a diet containing Bte and then fed these larvae to adult staphylinid beetles (*Paederus alferii*). Predator longevity was not significantly affected and no difference was seen in acceptability to predators between untreated larvae and those exposed to Bte.

Salama et al. (1982) treated aphids with sprays of Bte and provided these treated insects to newly hatched coccinellid larvae (*Coccinella undecimpunctata*). The survival of larvae of predators was not affected by feeding on the treated prey. However, the duration of predator larval development was increased in the group treated with Bte and there was a definite reduction in prey consumption.

Salama et al. (1982) evaluated the effect of Bte on the development of lacewing larvae (*Chrysopa carnea*) by presenting them with either sprayed aphids or treated cotton leafworm larvae (*Spodoptera littoralis*). When fed either the sprayed aphids or the treated cotton leafworms, the duration of larval development was significantly extended and prey consumption was significantly reduced.

6.4.2.3 *Honey-bees*

Krieg (1973) observed mortality in adult honey-bees (*Apis mellifera*) that were fed non-sporulated broth cultures of Btk. The mortalities were attributed to the thermolabile alpha-toxin. Since alpha-toxin is inactivated during sporulation, the toxin would not present a problem in sporulated commercial Btk products. When Krieg et al. (1980) fed fully sporulated cultures of Btk to adult honey-bees at concentrations of 1×10^8 spores and crystal per bee over a 7-day period, no harmful effects were observed.

Cantwell & Shieh (1981) fed a 1:20 solution of Btg in a sucrose solution to newly emerged adult honey-bees. After 14 days, there was no difference in mortality between treated and untreated groups. Treatment of hives resulted in no adverse effect on the adult workers or colony life as determined by egg laying, brood production, brood capping, or honey production.

Buckner et al. (1974) observed no adverse effects on honey-bees following aerial spraying of spruce (*Picea* species) with commercial Btk products.

Cantwell et al. (1966) fed honey-bees sugar solutions containing Btt spores, Btt culture supernatant with beta-exotoxin, and Btt crystals. The crystals did not harm the bees, but the supernatant caused nearly 100% mortality at day 7. Significant mortality was seen in the spore-treated bees at 8 days and was attributed to bacterial septicaemia. It should be noted that the dosages of each treatment were many times higher than the bees would be exposed to in the course of a lepidopteran control programme. Krieg (1973) reported mortality in honey-bees fed whole nonsporulated cultures of Btt, which was attributed to the presence of beta-exotoxin. Krieg & Herfs (1963) reported that vegetative cells of Btt did not harm honey-bees; however, they reported toxicity in Btt preparations containing the beta-exotoxin. Martouret & Euverte (1964) fed worker honey-bees cultures of Btt incorporated into mixtures of sugar, honey and clay. Complete mortality was seen at 7 days for the spore-crystal-exotoxin preparation and at 14 days for the spore-crystal complex.

6.4.2.4 Parasitoids

a) *Btk*

Dunbar & Johnson (1975) collected adult parasitoids (*Cardiochiles nigriceps*) in the field and fed them suspensions of a commercial Btk product. In the group fed Btk, shorter life spans were reported. Since the investigators could not be sure whether feeding actually took place, starvation may have been the cause of death.

Hassan & Krieg (1975) observed no adverse effects on adult chalcid wasps (*Trichogramma cacoeciae*) that were fed suspensions of a commercial Btk product. Krieg et al. (1980) fed washed spores and crystals of Btk (5×10^7 spores and crystals) for 7 days to adult chalcid wasps (*Trichogramma cacoeciae*) and observed no mortality or reduced capacity to parasitize.

Mück et al. (1981) reported significant mortality in adult braconids (*Cotesia glomerata*) that were fed a commercial Btk product at rates of 10^8 and 10^9 spores per ml, but observed little effect on the adult parasitoids (*Pimpla turionellae*). They reported midgut epithelial damage in the *Pimpla turionellae*, which resulted from the ICP.

Thomas & Watson (1986) found lower survival in adult ichneumonids (*Hyposoter exiguae*) fed suspensions of a commercial Btk product. They concluded the mortality was due to the spore-crystal complex.

Wallner & Surgeoner (1974) observed no effect on parasitoids following treatments with commercial Btk products for control of the notodontid moth (*Heterocampa manteo*).

Wallner et al. (1983) reported an indirect effect on the braconid *Rogas lymantriae* when it parasitized gypsy moth (*Lymantria dispar*) hosts fed Btk. The sex ratio of the parasitoid offspring was skewed towards males in the treated larvae, as the female parasitoids lay more fertilized eggs in larger, untreated host larvae.

Weseloh & Andreadis (1982) reported synergism in laboratory tests with gypsy moth larvae (*Lymantria dispar*) fed a commercial Btk product and exposed to the braconid (*Cotesia melanoscelus*). The percentage of parasitism was increased in Btk-intoxicated larvae since these grew more slowly and were at the approximate size suitable for parasitism for a longer time.

Buckner et al. (1974) reported no detrimental effects on parasitoid populations following field application of a commercial Btk product.

Dunbar et al. (1972) reported an increase in the percentage of parasitism of gypsy moth (*Lymantria dispar*) and elm spanworm (*Ennomos subsignarius*) larvae in forestry plots treated with a commercial Btk product.

Fusco (1980) reported an increase in the percentage of parasitism of gypsy moth (*Lymantria dispar*) larvae by the braconids *Cotesia melanoscelus* and *Phobocampe unicincta* following aerial sprays with a commercial Btk product.

Hamel (1977) found that parasitoids attacking early instar western spruce budworm larvae (*Choristoneura occidentalis*) increased in number following aerial application of a commercial Btk product, while older budworm larvae were reduced in number.

In two field studies, commercial Btk products showed no detrimental effects on parasitoid populations (Morris et al., 1977, 1980).

Wallner & Surgeoner (1974) demonstrated 6- to 12-fold increases in the percentage of parasitism in gypsy moth larvae (*Lymantria dispar*) by the braconid *Cotesia melanoscelus* in forestry plots treated with a commercial Btk product.

b) *Btt*

Hassan (1983) observed the chalcid *Trichogramma cacoeciae* was not affected by exposure to dried surface films of Btt.

Hassan & Krieg (1975) fed a suspension of three different commercial Bt products to adult chalcids (*Trichogramma cacoeciae*) and reported a minor reduction in the capacity to parasitize with Btt, but none with the other Bt products. The effect of the Btt product may have been due to the beta-exotoxin.

Krieg et al. (1980) fed washed spores and crystals of Btt to adult chalcids (*Trichogramma cacoeciae*) for 7 days and observed no mortality or reduced capacity to parasitize.

Lowered reproductive potential was observed for both the braconids *Microplitis demolitor* and *Zele chlorophthalma* following exposure to Btt (Salama et al., 1982; Salama & Zaki, 1983).

Salama & Zaki (1983) reported increased development times for *Zele chlorophthalma* parasitizing the cotton leafworm *Spodoptera littoralis* treated with Bte.

7. EXPOSURE AND EFFECTS ON HUMANS

There are some case reports on the occurrence of Bt in patients with different infectious diseases. However, none of these studies demonstrate an actual risk to human health by the use of Bt. They emphasize the need for further research on the production of toxins, knowledge of factors causing the genes of the toxins to be expressed, and knowledge on the natural occurrence of Bt and Bc. The medical practice does not discriminate between Bt and Bc as causative agents in infectious diseases. Therefore, the true proportion of Bt in Bc-induced disease is not known.

7.1 *Bacillus thuringiensis*

For aeons, humans have been exposed to Bt in their natural habitats, particularly from soil, water and the phylloplane. However in the recorded scientific literature, only few adverse effects to these environmental Bt levels have been documented.

The manufacture and field application of Bt products can result in aerosol and dermal exposure of workers and the human population, especially by spraying programmes in populated areas. Agricultural and horticultural uses of Bt can also result in dietary exposure.

7.1.1 *Experimental exposure of humans*

Eight human volunteers ingested 1 gram of a Btk formulation (3×10^9 spores/g of powder) daily for 5 days. Of the eight volunteers, five also inhaled 100 mg of the Btk powder daily for five days. Comprehensive medical examinations immediately before, after, and 4 to 5 weeks later failed to demonstrate any adverse health effects, and all the blood chemistry and urinalysis tests were negative (Fisher & Rosner, 1959).

Pivovarov et al. (1977) reported that ingestion of foods contaminated with Btg at concentrations of 10^5 to 10^9 cells/g caused nausea, vomiting, diarrhoea and tenesmus, colic-like pains in the abdomen, and fever in three of the four volunteers studied. The toxicity of the Btg strain may have been due to beta-exotoxin (Ray, 1990).

7.1.2. Exposure of workers during manufacture

Many manufacturers of Bt products monitor the exposure and the associated health risks of their workers. Over a period of 30 years of production, there have been no reports of such workers having been adversely affected (RJ Cibulsky, personal communication, 1997).

7.1.3 Exposure of workers in spraying operations

Noble et al. (1992) studied aerosol Btk exposure and subsequent nose and throat carriage of Bt by workers during a major spray programme for gypsy moth (*Lymantria dispar*) control. Spraying down from high lifts, spraying low foliage or spraying with prevailing breezes resulted in lower exposures of spray operators than did spraying upwards into trees. The mean exposure values ranged from 3.0×10^3 to 5.9×10^6 Bt spores/m^3 sampled air. Individuals working most shifts during the spray period were exposed to 5.4×10^6 to 7.2×10^7 organisms. Nearly all the workers exposed to higher concentrations for several shifts (5 to 20) were culture-positive for Bt, and the majority of the workers remained culture-positive for 14 to 30 days. Of those who were culture-positive, eight workers reverted to a culture-negative status during the project or within 30 days of project completion. During the spray programme, some workers experienced chapped lips, dry skin, eye irritation, and nasal drip and stuffiness, but no serious health problems resulted. These symptoms were transient and frequently occurred during the beginning of a spray run and when Bt spray concentrations were increased. No significant differences were found with respect to gender or smoking status.

In the same study, Noble et al. (1992) evaluated the health records of the general population in the county where the Btk spray programme was conducted. After examining the records of 3500 hospital emergency room admissions, 1140 family practice patients, and over 400 bacterial cultures from 10 hospitals, no evidence for community illness or infections attributed to Btk could be documented.

Laferrière et al. (1987) demonstrated antibody titres in 11 of 107 workers exposed to Btk during a 2-year spraying period. By the middle of the spray operation, seven had developed titres to spore-crystal complexes, six to vegetative cells, and one to spores. Their titres tended to be low, but were higher in those exposed for a second year. Two months after the exposure ended, nine workers were retested. Of these workers, five had no detectable antibodies to the spore-crystal complexes, and four who had been among those with the highest titres against vegetative cells had significantly lower titres.

Elliott et al. (1988) measured the exposure of individual workers and other individuals within the spraying area on the day of application during an aerial Btk spray programme for gypsy moth (*Lymantria dispar*) control. Concentrations of spores were measured using personal air sampling devices. The concentration of spores ranged from 0 to 1.1×10^4 cfu/m^3 for individual workers, the highest concentration being incurred by a spray card checker who was in brief contact with the material. For non-working individuals, the average Bt exposure was 1.3×10^3 cfu/m^3. In the spray area, a general survey showed concentrations of 0 to 4.2×10^3 cfu/m^3.

7.1.4 Exposure of human populations by spraying operations over populated areas

Btk and Bti have been sprayed over populated areas in several countries, including the USA, Canada and New Zealand. Some of these applications have been followed by public health surveillance programmes. In general, no (or very few) harmful effects have been reported among residents of the sprayed communities.

7.1.5 Clinical case reports

Commercial Bt products have been used for over two decades, but Bt has been isolated in only a few cases of human bacterial infection.

Samples & Buettner (1983) reported that a farm worker developed a corneal ulcer in one eye. It had been accidentally splashed with a commercial Btk product and Bt was subsequently isolated from the affected eye. The eye was treated with a topical antibiotic and corticosteroid and the corneal ulcer resolved 14 days after treatment. The report attributed the corneal ulcer to Bt infection. However, the possibility that Bt may have been a non-pathogenic contaminant of the ulcer was not considered. There are no other reports of Bt being associated with ocular infections in workers.

During the investigation of a gastroenteritis outbreak in a chronic care institution, bacteria were isolated from four individuals and were identified as B. *thuringiensis*. The Bt isolates showed cytotoxic effects characteristic of *B. cereus* (Jackson et al., 1995).

Damgaard et al. (1997a) isolated Bt in burn wounds in two patients. None of the isolates showed any toxicity to Vero cells. Hernandez et al. (1998) isolated Bt from a war wound; this strain (Bt *konkukian*) could infect immunosuppressed mice after cutaneous application.

Warren et al. (1984) reported that a research worker developed a marked local reaction and lymphadenitis following a needle stick injury when handling Bti. *Acinetobacter calcoaceticus* and Bt were cultured from the exudate. The condition responded to penicillin.

Green et al. (1990) reported that Bt was isolated from body fluids of 55 patients with different infectious diseases. In 52 of them, it was considered a contaminant, while in three cases with pre-existing medical problems, no firm conclusion was established concerning a causal relationship between the infection and Bt. Furthermore, Bt was isolated from the conjunctiva of a worker presenting with conjunctivitis, and with a history of a splash with a Bt product.

Despite the widespread use of Bt-based products, only two incidents of possible allergic reactions have been reported to the US EPA (McClintock et al., 1995). After detailed analysis, neither of these was considered to be causally related to Bt.

7.1.6 Dietary exposure of the general population

In some Asian countries, Bti has been added to domestic containers of drinking-water for mosquito control. From these high Bt exposures in drinking-water, no adverse effects in humans have been reported. In Africa, some rivers have been dosed with Bti at weekly intervals for blackfly control. No adverse effects in the human populations that drink the river water have been reported. Btk has been reported to survive for 1 to 2 months in fresh water and in seawater. However, viable Bt cultures have not been isolated from drinking-water supplies (Menon & De Mestral, 1985).

There is little information on levels of Bt to be found in food, but it is possible that, in view of the widespread prevalence of Bt, its presence in food is common and is not always related to its use on food products. Bt spores have been shown to be unable to germinate in mammalian digestive systems; however, Bt has been isolated from faecal and urinary samples in occupational studies.

Noble et al. (1992) reported that 5 out of 10 vegetable samples were positive for Btk. The positive samples were obtained from both supermarkets and from organically grown products. Such results may account for the recovery of Bt from faecal and urinary samples during the occupational studies and may reflect community exposure through food.

7.2 *Bacillus cereus*

The close affiliation between Bt and Bc raises the question of whether strains of Bt can cause human illness during vegetative growth. During vegetative growth Bc can produce different kinds of toxins; these toxins can cause gastrointestinal diseases in humans after ingestion. The emetic toxin is an enzymatically synthesized peptide that causes vomiting (Granum, 1997) a few hours after ingestion. Most Bc strains producing this toxin seem to belong to the same serotype (Mikami et al., 1995; Nishikawa et al., 1996). The enterotoxins are a group of proteins causing abdominal pain and diarrhoea after an incubation period of 8–16 h. The enterotoxins causing gastrointestinal disease are most likely produced in the small intestine. Characteristics of the two types of disease caused by Bc are shown Table 15. Based on analysis of outbreaks the infective dose is believed to vary between 10^5 and 10^8 vegetative cells or activated spores per gram, but it may be so low as 10^4 (Granum, 1997). In addition to the two toxins, Bc can produce different lytic enzymes, e.g., haemolysins, which most likely are involved in the gastrointestinal diseases. In addition to gastrointestinal diseases Bc can cause various diseases, notably in immunosuppressed individuals (Drobniewski, 1993).

Analysis of reported foodborne diseases reveals that Bc is frequently diagnosed as the cause of gastrointestinal disorders (Notermans & Batt, 1998) in many countries. Several food-borne disease outbreaks caused by Bc have been reported by Notermans & Batt (1998). However, Bc gastrointestinal diseases are highly under-

Table 15. Characteristics of the two types of disease caused by *B. cereus* (from Granum, 1997)

Characteristic	Emetic syndrome	Diarrhoeal
Infective dose (cells/g)	10^5–10^8	10^4–10^7
Toxin produced	Preformed in food	In the small intestine
Type of toxin	Cyclic peptide	Protein
Incubation period (h)	0.5–5	8–16 (occasionally >24)
Duration of illness	6–24	12–24 (occasionally many days)
Symptoms	Vomiting, nausea, malaise	Abdominal pain, diarrhoea

reported, as both types of illness are relatively mild and usually last less than 24 h (Granum, 1997; Notermans & Batt, 1998). The incidence of Bc in foods varies between 10^1 and 10^7, the highest concentrations being found in herbs/spices and boiled rice (Notermans & Batt, 1998). The degree of toxicity of enterotoxins varies from Bc strain to strain, probably due to differences in toxin components (Lund & Granum, 1997). Hassan & Nabbut (1996) found that clinical Bc isolates from human diarrhoeal faeces were strong producers of diarrhoeal enterotoxin, while isolates from blood, wounds, normal faeces, milk and rice were weak producers of diarrhoeal enterotoxin (Hassan & Nabbut, 1996). This variation is reflected in the variable numbers (10^5–10^8 viable cells or spores per g) of Bc reported to cause symptoms in humans, and it has been suggested that foods containing more than 10^4 Bc per g may not be safe for consumption (Granum, 1997). Several European countries have a critical level of 10^4–10^5 Bc per g for acceptance of food products (Notermans & Batt, 1998). This critical level will include Bt, as the methods used do not discriminate between Bc and Bt.

8. EVALUATION OF HUMAN HEALTH RISKS AND EFFECTS ON THE ENVIRONMENT

Owing to their specific mode of action, Bt products are unlikely to pose any hazard to humans or other vertebrates or to the great majority of non-target invertebrates provided that they are free from non-Bt microorganisms and from biologically active products other than the ICPs. Bt products may be safely used for the control of insect pests of agricultural and horticultural crops as well as forests. Bt is also safe for use in aquatic environments including drinking-water reservoirs for the control of mosquito, black fly and nuisance insect larvae. However, it should be noted that vegetative Bt have the potential for the production of Bc-like toxins, the significance of which as a cause of human disease is not known.

9. CONCLUSIONS AND RECOMMENDATIONS

- Bt may be safely used for the control of insect pests of agricultural crops and forests.

- Bti is safe for use in aquatic environments, including drinking-water reservoirs, for the control of mosquito, blackfly and nuisance insect larvae.

- Bt products should contain the ICPs and be free from other microorganisms and biologically active metabolites.

- New Bt products based on either new Bt strains and/or new ICPs require appropriate assessment.

- FAO and WHO should develop standard specifications for Bt preparations as is done for chemical pesticides.

- Good industrial large-scale practice (GILSP) standards should be employed for the production of Bt products.

- Standardized valid methods for the assessment of gastrointestinal consequences of vegetatively produced agents should be developed.

- The occurrence of resistant insect populations underscores the need for research on the relationships between *cry*-toxins and the ecology of Bt.

- More research on the fate of Bt spores and ICPs in the environment is needed. This should cover the natural occurrence of Bt and Bc in foods and its relationship to exposure to Bt from its pesticide use.

- Research into dose–response analysis and the consequent acceptable daily intake levels of Bt in the diet and beverages is a high priority.

10. PREVIOUS EVALUATIONS BY INTERNATIONAL ORGANISATIONS

WHO (1985) considered the safe use of MPCA at the Ninth Meeting of the WHO Expert Committee on Vector Control in 1984. The report considered that addition of live microorganisms to drinking-water is undesirable and recommended that the use of Bt H-14 for the control of *Aedes aegypti* in drinking-water should be restricted to the asporogenic form. At the 1990 meeting, WHO (1991), after reviewing new research data, stated that its previous recommendation was unduly restrictive, provided that properly designed formulations were used.

REFERENCES

Addison JA (1993) Persistence and nontarget effects of *Bacillus thuringiensis* in soil: a review. Can J Forensic Res, **23**: 2329–2342.

Agata N, Ohta M, Arakawa Y, & Mori M (1995) The *bceT* gene of *Bacillus cereus* encodes an enterotoxic protein. Microbiology, **141**: 983–988.

Ahmed R, Sankar-Mistry P, Jackson S, Ackermann H-W, & Kasatiya SS (1995) *Bacillus cereus* phage typing as an epidemiological tool in outbreaks of food poisoning. J Clin Microbiol, **33**: 636–640.

Akiba Y (1986) Microbial ecology of *Bacillus thuringiensis*: VI. Germination of *Bacillus thuringiensis* spores in the soil. Appl Entomol Zool, **21**: 76–80.

Akiba Y (1991) Assessment of rainwater-mediated dispersion of field-sprayed *Bacillus thuringiensis* in the soil. Appl Entomol Zool, **26**: 477–483.

Ali A (1980) Nuisance chironomids and their control: a review. Bull Entomol Soc Am, **26**: 3–16.

Ali A (1981) *Bacillus thuringiensis* serovar. *israelensis* (ABG-6108) against chironomids and some nontarget aquatic invertebrates. J Invertebr Pathol, **38**: 264–272.

Ali A & Baggs RD (1981) Susceptibility of some Florida chironomids and mosquitoes to various formulations of *Bacillus thuringiensis* serovar *israelensis de Barjac*. J Econ Entomol, **74**: 672–677.

Aly C (1985) Germination of *Bacillus thuringiensis* var. *israelensis* spores in the gut of *Aedes* larvae (Diptera: Culicidae). J Invertebr Pathol, **45**: 1–8.

Aly C & Mulla MS (1987) Effect of two microbial insecticides on aquatic predators of mosquitoes. J Appl Entomol, **103**: 113–118.

Aly C, Mulla MS, & Federici BA (1985) Sporulation and toxin production by *Bacillus thuringiensis* var. *israelensis* in cadavers of mosquito larvae (Diptera: Culicidae). J Invertebr Pathol, **46**: 251–258.

Andersson MA, Mikkola R, Helin J, Andersson MC, & Salkinoja-Salonen M (1998) A novel sensitive bioassay for detection of *Bacillus cereus* emetic toxin and related depsipeptide ionophores. Appl Environ Microbiol, **64**: 1338–1343.

Andrews RE Jr, Faust RM, Wabiko H, Raymond KC, & Bulla LA Jr (1987) The biotechnology of *Bacillus thuringiensis*. CRC Crit Rev Biotechnol, **6**: 163–232.

Angus TA (1954) A bacterial toxin paralysing silkworm larvae. Nature (Lond), **173**: 545–546.

Aronson AI, Han ES, McGaughey W, & Johnson D (1991) The solubility of inclusion proteins from *Bacillus thuringiensis* is dependent upon protoxin composition and is a factor in toxicity to insects. Appl Environ Microbiol, **57**: 981–986.

Asano S-I, Nukumizu Y, Bando H, Hzuka T, & Yamamoto T (1997) Cloning of novel enterotoxin genes from *Bacillus cereus* and *Bacillus thuringiensis*. Appl Environ Microbiol, **63**: 1054–1057.

Ash C, Farrow JA, Dorsch M, Stackebrandt E, & Collins MD (1991) Comparative analysis of *Bacillus anthracis*, *Bacillus cereus*, and related species on the basis of reverse transcriptase sequencing of 16S rRNA. Int J System Bacteriol, **41**: 343-346.

Asquith D (1975) Response of the predaceous black lady beetle *Stethorus punctum* (DeConte) to apple orchard insecticide treatments (Experiment No. D986-4007). Chicago, Illinois, Abbott Laboratories.

Baida GE & Kuzmin NP (1995) Cloning and primary structure of a new hemolysin gene from *Bacillus cereus*. Biochim Biophys Acta, **1264**: 151–154.

Baumann L, Okamoto K, Unterman BM, Lynch MJ, & Bauman P (1984) Phenotypic characterization of *Bacillus thuringiensis* and *Bacillus cereus*. J Invertebr Pathol, **44**: 329–341.

Beach RM (1990) Application for an experimental use permit to ship and use a pesticide for experimental purposes only — Permit No. 58788-EUP-4 for InCide[M] 586. Hanover, Maryland, Crop Genetics International.

Beattie SH, Holt C, Hirst D, & Williams AG (1998) Discrimination among *Bacillus cereus, B. mycoides* and *B. thuringiensis* and some other species of the genus *Bacillus* by Fourier transform infrared spectroscopy. FEMS Microbiol Lett, **164**: 201–206.

Beavers JB (1991a) ABG-6305: An avian oral pathogenicity and toxicity study in the mallard (Project No. 161-118). Easton, Maryland, Wildife International Ltd, pp 1–20 (Unpublished Abbott document).

Beavers JB (1991b) ABG-6305: An avian oral pathogenicity and toxicity study in the bobwhite (Project No. 161-117). Easton, Maryland, Wildife International Ltd, pp 1–21 (Unpublished Abbott document).

Beavers JB, Larsen AC, & Jaber M (1989a) *Bacillus thuringiensis* var. *tenebrionis*: An avian single dose oral toxicity and pathogenicity study in the bobwhite (Project No. 161-109). Eston, Maryland, Wildlife International Ltd, pp 1–19 (Unpublished Abbott document).

Beavers JB, Clauss BS, & Jaber M (1989b) *Bacillus thuringiensis* var. *tenebrionis*: An avian single dose oral toxicity and pathogenicity study in the mallard (Project No. 161-108). Easton, Maryland, Wildlife International Ltd, pp 1–19 (Unpublished Abbott document).

Becker N & Margalit J (1993) Use of *Bacillus thuringiensis israelensis* against mosquitoes and blackflies. In: Entwistle PF, Cory JS, Bailey MJ, & Higgs S ed. *Bacillus thuringiensis*, an environmental biopesticide: Theory and practice. Chichester, New York, Toronto, Wiley & Sons, pp 147–170.

Beegle CC, Dulmage HT, Wolfenbarger DA, & Martinez E (1981) Persistence of *Bacillus thuringiensis* Berliner insecticidal activity on cotton foliage. Environ Entomol, **10**: 400–401.

Benz G & Altwegg A (1975) Safety of *Bacillus thuringiensis* for earthworms. J Invertebr Pathol, **26**: 125–126.

Berliner E (1915) [About the sleep sickness of the *Ephestia kühniella Zell.* and its vector *Bacillus thuringiensis.*] Z Angew Entomol, **2:** 29–56 (in German).

Bernhard K & Utz R (1993) Production of *Bacillus thuringiensis* insecticides for experimental and commercial uses. In: Entwistle PF, Cory JS, Bailey MJ, & Higgs S ed. *Bacillus thuringiensis*, an environmental biopesticide: Theory and practice. Chichester, New York, Toronto, Wiley & Sons, pp 255–267.

Bernier RL Jr, Gannon DJ, Moser GP, Mazzarello M, Griffiths MM, & Guest PJ (1990) Development of a novel Bt strain for the control of forestry pests. In: Brighton Crop Protection Conference — Pests and Diseases — 1990: Proceedings. Farnham, Surrey, British Crop Protection Council, pp 245–252.

Boeri RL (1991) Acute toxicity of ABG-6305 to the rainbow trout (*Oncorhynchus mykiss*) (Project No. 9107-A). Hampton, New Hampshire, Resource Analysts Inc, Enviro Systems Division, pp 1–26 (Unpublished Abbott document).

Bonnefoi A & Béguin S (1959) Recherches sur l'action des cristaux de *Bacillus thuringiensis* souche "anduze". Entomophaga, **4**: 193–199.

Bourque SN, Valero JR, Lavoie MC, & Levesque RC (1995) Comparative analysis of the 16S-23S ribosomal intergenic spacer sequences of *Bacillus thuringiensis* strains and subspecies and of closely related species. Appl Environ Microbiol, **61**: 1623–1626.

Bravo A, Sarabia S, Lopez L, Ontiveros H, Abarca C, Ortiz M, Lina L, Villalobos FJ, Pena G, Nunez-Valdez M-E, Soberón M, & Quintero R (1998) Characterization of *cry* genes in a Mexican *Bacillus thuringienis* strain collection. Appl Environ Microbiol, **64**: 4965–4972.

Brousseau R, Saint-Onge A, Prefontaine G, Masson L, & Cabana J (1992) Arbitrary primer polymerase chain reaction, a powerful method to identify *Bacillus thuringiensis* serovars and strains. Appl Environ Microbiol, **59**: 114–119.

Buckner CH, Kingsbury PD, McLeod BB, Mortensen KL, & Ray DGH (1974) Impact of aerial treatment on non-target organisms, Algonquin Park, Ontario, and Spruce Woods, Manitoba, Section F. In: Evaluation of commercial preparations of *Bacillus thuringiensis* with and without chitinase against spruce budworm. Ottawa, Ontario, Canadian Forestry Service, Chemial Control Research Institute, pp 1–72 (Information report CC-X-59).

Bulla LA Jr, Kramer KJ, & Davidson LI (1977) Characterization of the entomocidal parasporal crystal of *Bacillus thuringiensis*. J Bacteriol, **130**: 375–383.

Bulla LA Jr, Faust RM, Andrews R, & Goodman N (1985) Insecticidal bacilli. In: Dubnau DA ed. The molecular biology of the bacilli. New York, London, Academic Press Inc., vol 2, pp 185–209.

Burges HD (1977) Control of the wax moth *Galleria mellonella* on beecomb by H-serotype V *Bacillus thuringiensis* and the effect of chemical additives. Apidologie, **8**: 155–168.

Burges HD (1980) Safety, safety testing and quality control of microbial pesticides. In: Burges HD ed. Microbial control of pests and plant diseases 1970–1980. New York, London, Academic Press Inc., pp 738–767.

Burges HD & Bailey L (1968) Control of the greater and lesser wax moths (*Galleria mellonella* and *Achroia griesella*) with *Bacillus thuringiensis*. J Invertebr Pathol, **11**: 184–195.

Burges HD & Hurst JA (1977) Ecology of *Bacillus thuringiensis* in storage moths. J Invertebr Pathol, **30**: 131–139.

Calamari D, Yameogo L, Hougard J-M, & Levêque C (1998) Environmental assessment of larvicide use in the onchocerciasis control programme. Parasitol Today, **14**: 485–489.

Campbell DP, Dieball DE, & Brackett JM (1987) Rapid HPLC assay for the ß-exotoxin of *Bacillus thuringiensis*. J Agric Food Chem, **35**: 156–158.

Cannon RJC (1996) *Bacillus thuringiensis* use in agriculture: a molecular perspective. Biol Rev Cambridge Philos Soc, **71**: 561–636.

Cantwell GE & Shieh TR (1981) Certan™: A new bacterial insecticide against the greater wax moth. Am Bee J, **121**: 424–431.

Cantwell GE, Heimpel AM, & Thompson MJ (1964) The production of an exotoxin by various crystal-forming bacteria related to *Bacillus thuringiensis* var. *thuringiensis* Berliner. J Insect Pathol, **6**: 466–480.

Cantwell GE, Knox DA, Lehnert T, & Michael AS (1966) Mortality of the honey bee *Apis mellifera*, in colonies treated with certain biological insecticides. J Invertebr Pathol, **8**: 228–233.

Car M (1984) Laboratory and field trials with two *Bacillus thuringiensis* var. *israelensis* products for *Simulium* (Diptera: Nematocera) control in a small polluted river in South Africa. Onderstepoort J Vet Res, **51**: 141–144.

Car M & de Moor FC (1984) The response of Vaal River drift and benthos to *Simulium* (Diptera: Nematocera) control using *Bacillus thuringiensis* var. *israelensis* (H-14). Onderstepoort J Vet Res, **51**: 155–160.

Carlberg G, Kihamia CM, & Minhar J (1985) Mcrobial control of flies in latrines in Dar es Salaam with a *Bacillus thuringiensis* (serotype 1) preparation, Muscabac. J Appl Microbiol Biotechnol, **1**: 33–44.

Carlson CR & Kolstø A-B (1993) A complete physical map of a *Bacillus thuringiensis* chromosome. J Bacteriol, **175**: 1053–1060.

Carlson CR, Caugant DA, & Kolstr A-B (1994) Genotypic diversity among *Bacillus cereus* and *Bacillus thuringiensis* strains. Appl Environ Microbiol, **60**: 1719–1725.

Carlton BC, Gawron-Burke C, & Johnson TB (1990) Exploiting the genetic diversity of *Bacillus thuringiensis* for the creation of new bioinsecticides. In: Proceedings of the 5th International Colloquium on Invertebrate Pathology and Microbial Control. Adelaide, Australia, Society for Invertebrate Pathology, pp 18–22.

Chilcott CN, Pillai JS, & Kalmakoff J (1983) Efficacy of *Bacillus thuringiensis* var. *israelensis* as a biocontrol agent against larvae of Simuliidae (Diptera) in New Zealand. NZ J Zool, **10**: 319–326.

Christensen KP (1990a) Dipel technical material (*Bacillus thuringiensis* var. *kurstaki*): Infectivity and pathogenicity to bluegill sunfish (*Lepomis macrochirus*) during a 32-day static renewal test. Wareham, Massachusetts, Springborn Laboratories Inc., pp 1–53 (Unpublished Abbott document No. 90-1-3211).

Christensen KP (1990b) Dipel technical material (*Bacillus thuringiensis* var. *kurstaki*): Infectivity and pathogenicity to rainbow trout (*Oncorhynchus mykiss*) during a 32-day static renewal test.

Wareham, Massachusetts, Springborn Laboratories Inc., pp 1–57(Unpublished Abbott document No. 90-2-3219).

Christensen KP (1990c) Dipel technical material (*Bacillus thuringiensis* var. *kurstaki*): Infectivity and pathogenicity to sheepshead minnow (*Cyprinodon variegatus*) during a 30-day static renewal test. Wareham, Massachusetts, Springborn Laboratories Inc., vol 2, pp 253–308 (Unpublished Abbott document No. 90-5-3317).

Christensen KP (1990d) *Bacillus thuringiensis* var. *tenebrionis*: Infectivity and pathogenicity to rainbow trout (*Oncorhynchus mykiss*) during a 30-day static renewal test. Wareham, Massachusetts, Springborn Laboratories Inc., pp 1–54 (Unpublished Abbott document No. 90-3-3263).

Christensen KP (1990e) *Bacillus thuringiensis* var. *tenebrionis*: Infectivity and pathogenicity to sheepshead minnow (*Cyprinodon variegatus*) during a 30-day static renewal test. Wareham, Massachusetts, Springborn Laboratories Inc., pp 1–50 (Unpublished Abbott document No. 90-6-3348).

Christensen KP (1990f) Vectobac technical material (*Bacillus thuringiensis* var. *israelensis*): Infectivity and pathogenicity to bluegill sunfish (*Lepomis macrochirus*) during a 30-day static renewal test. Wareham, Massachusetts, Springborn Laboratories Inc., pp 1–55 (Unpublished Abbott document No. 90-2-3228).

Christensen KP (1990g) Vectobac technical material (*Bacillus thuringiensis* var. *israelensis*): Infectivity and pathogenicity to rainbow trout (*Oncorhynchus mykiss*) during a 32-day static renewal test. Wareham, Massachusetts, Springborn Laboratories Inc., pp 1–55 (Unpublished Abbott document No. 90-2-3242).

Christensen KP (1990h) Vectobac technical material (*Bacillus thuringiensis* var. *israelensis*): Infectivity and pathogenicity to sheepshead minnow (*Cyprinodon variegatus*) during a 30-day static renewal test. Wareham, Massachusetts, Springborn Laboratories Inc., pp 1–57 (Unpublished Abbott document No. 90-4-3288).

Cibulsky RJ & Fusco RA (1987) Recent experiences with Vectobac for black fly control: An industrial perspective on future developments. In: Kim KC & Merritt RW ed. Black flies: Ecology, population management, and annotated world list. University Park, Pennsylvania, Pennsylvania State University Press, pp 419–424.

Claus D & Berkeley RCW (1986) Genus *Bacillus* Cohn 1872. In: Sneath PHA, Mair NS, Sharp ME, & Holt JG ed. Bergey's manual of systematic bacteriology. Baltimore, Maryland, Williams& Wilkins, vol 2, pp 1105–1139.

Cooksey KE (1971) The protein crystal toxin of *Bacillus thuringiensis*: Biochemistry and mode of action. In: Burges HD & Hussey NW ed. Microbial control of insects and mites. New YorkLondon, Academic Press Inc., pp 247–274.

Crickmore N, Zeigler DR, Feitelson J, Schnepf E, van Rie J, Lereclus D, Baum J, & Dean DH (1998) Revision of the nomenclature for the *Bacillus thuringiensis* pesticidal crystal proteins. Microbiol Mol Biol Rev, **62**: 807–813.

Damgaard PH (1995) Diarrhoeal enterotoxin production by strains of *Bacillus thuringiensis* isolated from commercial *Bacillus thuringiensis* — based insecticides. FEMS Immunol Med Microbiol, **12**: 245–250.

Damgaard PH, Granum PE, Bresciani J, Torregrossa MV, Eilenberg J, & Valentino L (1997a) Characterization of *Bacillus thuringiensis* isolated from infections in burn wounds. FEMS Immunol Med Microbiol, **18**: 47–53.

Damgaard PH, Hansen BM, Pedersen JC, & Eilenberg J (1997b) Natural occurrence of *B. thuringiensis* on cabbage foliage and in insects associated with cabbage crops. J Appl Bacteriol, **82**: 253–258.

Damgaard PH, Larsen HD, Hansen BM, Bresciani J, & Jørgensen K (1996a) Enterotoxin-producing strains of *Bacillus thuringiensis* isolated from food. Lett Appl Microbiol, **23**: 146–150.

Damgaard PH, Jacobsen CS, & Sørensen J (1996b) Development and application of a primer set for specific detection of *Bacillus thuringiensis* and *Bacillus cereus* in soil using magnetic capture-hybridization and PCR amplification. System Appl Microbiol, **19**: 436–441.

de Barjac H (1981a) Identification of H-serotypes of *Bacillus thuringiensis*. In: Burges HD ed. Microbial control of pests and plant diseases 1970–1980. New York, London, Academic Press Inc., pp 35–43.

de Barjac H (1981b) Insect pathogens in the genus *Bacillus*. In: Berkley RCW & Goodfellow M ed. The aerobic endospore-forming bacteria: Classification and identification. New York, London, Academic Press Inc., pp 241–250.

de Barjac H & Bonnefoi A (1962) Essai de classification biochimique et sérologique de 24 souches de *Bacillus* de type *thuringiensis*. Entomophaga, **7**: 5–31.

de Barjac H & Larget-Thiery I (1984) Characteristics of IPS 82 as standard for biological assays of *Bacillus thuringiensis* H-14 preparations. Geneva, World Health Organization (WHO/VBC/84.892).

de Barjac H, Larget I, Bénichou L, Cosmao V, Viviani G, Ripouteau H, & Papion S (1980) Test d'innocuité sur mammifères avec du sérotype H 14 de *Bacillus thuringiensis*. Geneva, World Health Organization (WHO/VBC/80.761).

Dean DH (1984) Biochemical genetics of the bacterial insect-control agent *Bacillus thuringiensis*: Basic principles and prospects for genetic engineering. Biotechnol Genet Eng Rev, **2**: 341–363.

Dean DH, Rajamohan F, Lee MK, Wu SJ, Chen XJ, Alcantara E, & Hussain SR (1996) Probing the mechanism of action of *Bacillus thuringiensis* insecticidal proteins by site-directed mutagenesis – a minireview. Gene, **179**: 111–117.

DeLucca AJ II, Simonson JG, & Larson AD (1981) *Bacillus thuringiensis* distribution in soils of the United States. Can J Microbiol, **27**: 865–870.

Demezas DH & Bell J (1995) Evaluation of low molecular weight RNA profiles and ribotyping to differentiate some *Bacillus* species. System Appl Microbiol, **18**: 582–589.

Denolf P, Hendrickx K, Vandamme J, Jansens S, Peferoen M, Degheele D, & Vanrie J (1997) Cloning and characterization of *Manduca sexta* and *Plutella xylostella* midgut aminopeptidase N enzymes related to *Bacillus thuringiensis* toxin-binding proteins. Eur J Biochem, **248**: 748–761.

Dent DR (1993) The use of *Bacillus thuringiensis* as an insecticide. In: Jones DG ed. Exploitation of microorganisms. London, Chapman & Hall, pp 19–44.

Drobniewski FA (1993) *Bacillus cereus* and related species. Clin Microbiol Rev, **6**: 324-338.

Dulmage HT & cooperators (1981) Insecticidal activity of isolates of *Bacillus thuringiensis* and their potential for pest control. In: Burges HD ed. Microbial control of pests and plant diseases 1970–1980. New York, London, Academic Press Inc., pp 193–223.

Dunbar JP & Johnson AW (1975) *Bacillus thuringiensis*: Effects on the survival of a tobacco budworm parasitoid and predator in the laboratory. Environ Entomol, **4**: 352–354.

Dunbar DM, Kaya HK, Doane CC, Anderson JF, & Weseloh RM (1972) Aerial application of *Bacillus thuringiensis* against larvae of the elm spanworm and gypsy moth and effects on parasitoids of the gypsy moth. Connecticut Experiment Station (Bulletin No. 735).

Eilenberg J, Damgaard PH, Hansen BM, Pedersen JC, Bresciani J, & Larsson R (in press) Natural interactions between *Strongwellsea castrans*, *Cystosporogenes deliaradicae* and *Bacillus thuringiensis* in the host, *Delia radicum*. J Invertebr Pathol.

Elliott LJ, Sokolow R, Heumann M, & Elefant SL (1988), An exposure characterization of a large scale application of a biological insecticide, *Bacillus thuringiensis*. Appl Ind Hyg, **3**: 119–122.

Elsey KD (1973) *Jalysus spinosus* effect of insecticide treatments on this predator of tobacco pests. Environ Entomol, **2**: 240–243.

Entwistle PF, Cory JS, Bailey MJ, & Higgs S (1983) *Bacillus thuringiensis*, an environmental biopesticide: Theory and practice. Chichester, New York, Toronto, John Wiley & Sons, 311 pp.

Estruch JJ, Warren GW, Mullins MA, Nye GJ, Craig JA, & Koziel MG (1996) Vip3A, a novel *Bacillus thuringiensis* vegetative insecticidal protein with a wide spectrum of activities against lepidopteran insects. Proc Natl Acad Sci (USA), **93**: 5389–5394.

Farkaš J, Šebesta K, Horská K, Samek Z, Dolejš L, & Šorm F (1977) Structure of thuringiensin, the thermostable exotoxin from *Bacillus thuringiensis*. Coll Czech Chem Commun, **42**: 909–929.

Fast PG (1971) Isolation of a water-soluble toxin from a commercial microbial insecticide based on *Bacillus thuringiensis*. J Invertebr Pathol, **17**: 301.

Fast PG (1981) The crystal toxin of *Bacillus thuringiensis*. In: Burges HD ed. Microbial control of pests and plant diseases 1970–1980. New York, London, Academic Press Inc., pp 223–248.

Faust RM (1973) The *Bacillus thuringiensis* β-exotoxin: Current status. Bull Entomol Soc Am, **19**: 153–156.

Feitelson JS (1993) The *Bacillus thuringiensis* family tree. In: Kim L ed. Advanced engineered pesticides. New York, Basel, Marcel Dekker Inc., pp 63-71.

Fisher R & Rosner L (1959) Toxicology of the microbial insecticide, Thuricide. J Agric Food Chem, **7**: 686–688.

Frommer W, Ager B, Archer L, Brunius G, Collins CH, Donikian R, Frontali C, Hamp S, Houwink EH, Kuenzi MT, Krämer P, Lagast H, Lund S, Mahler JL, Normand-Plessier F, Sargeant K, Tuijnenburg-Muijs G, Vranch SP, & Werner RG (1989) Safe biotechnology: II. Safety precautions for handling microorganisms of different risk classes. Appl Microbiol Biotechnol, **30**: 541–552.

Fusco RA (1980) Field evaluation of a commercial preparation of *Bacillus thuringiensis*, DIPEL 4L: Progress report. Pennsylvania Bureau of Forestry, Gypsy Moth Pest Management Methods Development Project.

Gaddis PK & Corkran CC (1986) Secondary effects of Bt spray on avian predators: the reproductive success of chestnut-backed chickadees. Northwest Ecological Research Institute (Unpublished Research Report No. 86–03).

Garcia R, Des Rochers B, & Tozer W (1980) Studies on the toxicity of *Bacillus thuringiensis* var. *israelensis* against organisms found in association with mosquito larvae. Berkeley, California, University of California, Division of Biological Control.

Gelernter WD (1990) Targeting insecticide-resistant markets: New developments in microbial-based products. In: Green MB, Moberg WK, & LeBaron H ed. Managing resistance to agrochemicals: From fundamental research to practical strategies. Washington, DC, American Chemical Society, pp 105–117 (ACS Series 421).

Giffel MC, Beumer RR, Klijn N, Wagendorp A, & Rombouts FM (1997) Discrimination between *Bacillus cereus* and *Bacillus thuringiensis* using specific DNA probes based on variable regions of 16S rRNA. FEMS Microbiol Lett, **146**: 47–51.

Gill SS, Hornung JM, Ibarra JE, Singh GJP, & Federici BA (1987) Cytolytic activity and immunological similarity of *Bacillus thuringiensis* subsp. *israelensis* and *Bacillus thuringiensis* subsp. *morrisoni* isolate PG-14 toxins. Appl Environ Microbiol, **53**: 1251–1256.

Gilmore MS, Cruz-Rodz AL, Leimeister-Wächter M, Kreft J, & Goebel W (1989) A *Bacillus cereus* cytolytic determinant, cereolysin AB, which comprises the phospholipase C and sphingomyelinase genes: Nucleotide sequence and genetic linkage. J Bacteriol, **171**: 744–753.

Goldberg LJ & Margalit J (1977) A bacterial spore demonstrating rapid larvicidal activity against *Anopheles sergentii, Uranotaenia unguiculata, Culex univitattus, Aedes aegypti* and *Culex pipiens.* Mosq News, **37**: 355–358.

González JM Jr & Carlton BC (1980) Patterns of plasmid DNA in crystalliferous and acrystalliferous strains of *Bacillus thuringiensis*. Plasmid, **3**: 92–98.

González JM Jr, Dulmage HT, & Carlton BC (1981) Correlation between specific plasmids and δ-endotoxin production in *Bacillus thuringiensis*. Plasmid, **5**: 351–365.

González JM, Jr Brown BJ, & Carlton BC (1982) Transfer of *Bacillus thuringiensis* plasmids coding for δ-endotoxin among strains of *B. thuringiensis* and *B. cereus*. Proc Natl Acad Sci (USA), **79**: 6951–6955.

Gordon RE (1977) Some taxonomic observations on the genus *Bacillus*. In: Briggs JB ed. Biological regulations of vectors: The saprophytic and aerobic bacteria and fungi. Washington, DC, US Department of Health, Education and Welfare, pp 67–82 (Publication NIH 77-1180).

Granum PE (1997) *Bacillus cereus*. In: Doyle MP, Beuchat LR, & Montville TJ ed. Food microbiology fundamentals and frontiers. Washington, DC, ASM Press, pp 327–336.

Grassi S & Deseö KV (1984) [The natural occurrence of *Bacillus thuringiensis* Berl. And its importance in the plant protection.] In: [Proceedings of Seminar on Phytopathology, Sorrento, Italy 26–29 March 1984.] Bologna, Italy, Clueb Publishing Co., vol 2, pp 424–433 (in Italian).

Green M, Heumann M, Sokolow R, Foster LR, Bryant R, & Skeels M (1990) Public health implications of the microbial pesticide *Bacillus thuringiensis*: An epidemiological study, Oregon, 1985–1986. Am J Publ Health, **80**: 848–852.

Griego VM & Spence KD (1978) Inactivation of *Bacillus thuringiensis* spores by ultraviolet and visible light. Appl Environ Microbiol, **35**: 906–910.

Grochulski P, Masson L, Borisova S, Pusztai-Carey M, Schwartz JL, Brousseau R, & Cygler M (1995) *Bacillus thuringiensis* CryIA(a) insecticidal toxin: crystal structure and channel formation. J Mol Biol, **254**: 447–464.

Hadley WM, Burchiel SW, McDowell TD, Thilsted JP, Hibbs CM, Whorton JA, Day PW, Friedman MB, & Stoll RE (1987) Five-month oral (diet) toxicity/ infectivity study of *Bacillus thuringiensis* insecticides in sheep. Fundam Appl Toxicol, **8**: 236–242.

Hamed AR (1978–79) [Effects of *Bacillus thuringiensis* on parasites and predators of *Yponomeuta evenymellus* (Lep., Yponomeutidae).] Z Angew Entomol, **87**: 294–311 (in German).

Hamel DR (1977) The effects of *Bacillus thuringiensis* on parasitoids of the western spruce budworm, *Choristoneura occidentalis* (Lepidoptera: Tortricidae), and the spruce coneworm, *Dioryctria reniculelloides* (Lepidoptera: Pyralidae), in Montana. Can Entomol, **109**: 1409–1415.

Hannay CL (1953) Crystalline inclusions in aerobic spore-forming bacteria. Nature (Lond), **172**: 1004.

Hansen BM & Hendriksen NB (1997a) *Bacillus thuringiensis* and *B. cereus* enterotoxins: Proceedings of the 6th European Meeting of the International Organization for Biological and Integrated Control of Noxious Animals and Plants/West Paleaearctic Regional Section, Copenhagen, 10–15 August 1997. Copenhagen, Denmark, Royal Veterinary and Agricultural University, Department of Ecology and Molecular Biology.

Hansen BM & Hendriksen NB (1997b) Comparative PCR analysis of *B. thuringiensis* and *B. cereus*: Abstract for the International Workshop on Molecular Biology of *B. cereus*, *B. anthracis* and *B. thuringiensis*, Soria Moria, Oslo, 23–25 May 1997.

Hansen BM & Hendriksen NB (1999) Ecological aspects of the survival in soil of spray released *Bacillus thuringiensis* subsp. *kurstaki*. In: Abstract for the IOBC Symposium on Indirect Ecological Effects of Biological Control, Montpelier, 17–20 October 1999. Montpelier, France, Agropolis International.

Hansen BM, Damgaard PH, Eilenberg J, & Pedersen JC (1996) *Bacillus thuringiensis*, ecology and environmental effects of its use for microbial pest control (Environmental Project No. 316). Copenhagen, Denmark, Ministry of Environment and Energy, Danish Environmental Protection Agency.

Hansen BM, Damgaard PH, Eilenberg J, & Pedersen JC (1998) Molecular and phenotypic characterization of *Bacillus thuringiensis* isolated from leaves and insects. J Invertebr Pathol, **71**: 106–114.

Harding J, Wolfenbarger D, Dupnik T, & Fuchs T (1972) Large scale tests comparing *Bacillus thuringiensis* with methyl-parathion for cotton insect control, field test report. Chicago, Illinois, Abbott Laboratories (Unpublished document).

Hassan SA (1983) Results of laboratory testing of a series of pesticides on egg parasites of the genus *Trichogramma* (Hymenoptera, Trichogrammatidae). Nachr.bl Dtsch Pflanzenschutzdienstes (Braunschweig), **35**: 21.

Hassan S & Krieg A (1975) [*Bacillus thuringiensis* preparations harmless to the parasite *Trichogramma cacoeciae* (Hym.: Trichogrammatidae).] ZPflanzenkr Pflanzenchutz, **82**: 515–521 (in German).

Hassan G & Nabbut N (1996) Prevalence and characterization of*Bacillus cereus* isolates from clinical and natural sources. J Food Prot, **59**: 193–196.

Heimpel AM (1954) Investigations of the mode of action ofstrains of *Bacillus cereus* Frankland and Frankland pathogenic for the larch sawfly, *Pristiphora chrichsonii* (Htg.). Kingston, Canada, Queen's University, 155 pp (Doctoral dissertation).

Heimpel AM (1967) A critical review of*Bacillus thuringiensis* var. *thuringiensis* Berliner and other crystalliferous bacteria. Annu Rev Entomol, **12**: 287–322.

Heimpel AM & Angus TA (1958) The taxonomy of insect pathogens related to*Bacillus cereus* Frankland and Frankland. Can J Microbiol, **4**: 531–541.

Helgason E, Caugant DA, Lecadet M-M, Chen Y, Mahillon J, Lövgren A, Hegna I, Kvaløy K& Kolstø A-B (1998) Genetic diversity of *Bacillus cereus*/*B. thuringiensis* isolates from natural sources. Curr Microbiol, **37**: 80–87.

Hendriksen NB & Hansen BM (1998) Phylogenetic relations of*Bacillus thuringiensis*: Implications for risks associated to its use as a microbiological pest control agent. IOBC Bull, **21**: 5–8.

Hernandez E, Ramisse F, Ducoureau J-P, Cruel T, & Cavallo J-D (1998)*Bacillus thuringiensis* subsp. *konkukian* (serotype H34) superinfection: Case report and experimental evidence of pathogenicity in immunosuppressed mice. J Clin Microbiol, **36**: 2138–2139.

Höfte H & Whiteley HR (1989) Insecticidal crystal proteins of*Bacillus thuringiensis*. Microbiol Rev, **53**: 242–255.

Honée G & Visser B (1993) The mode of action of*Bacillus thuringiensis* crystal proteins. Entomol Exp Appl, **69**: 145–155.

Horn DJ (1983) Selective mortality of parasitoids and predators of*Myzus persicae* on collards treated with malathion, carbaryl, or *Bacillus thuringiensis*. Entomol Exp Appl, **34**: 208–211.

Horsburgh R & Cobb L (1981) Effect of Dipel WP and Dipel + Guthion tank mix combination for control of variegated leafroller, turfed apple bud moth, and red-banded leafroller larvae on apples in a full season and late season program in Virginia (Experiment No. D-986-4240). Chicago, Illinois, Abbott Laboratories Inc.

Hostetter DL, Ignoffo CM, & Kearby WH (1975) Persistence of formulations of *Bacillus thuringiensis* spores and crystals on eastern red cedar foliage in Missouri. J Kansas Entomol Soc, **48**: 189–193.

Hotha S & Banik RM (1997) Production of alkaline protease by *Bacillus thuringiensis* H 14 in aqueous two-phase systems. J Chem Technol Biotechnol, **69**: 5–10.

Huber HE & Lüthy P (1981) *Bacillus thuringiensis* delta-endotoxin: Composition and activation. In: Davidson EW ed. Pathogenesis of invertebrate microbial diseases. Totowa, New Jersey, Allanheld-Osmun Publishers, pp 209–234.

Huber HE, Lüthy P, Ebersold HR, & Cordier JL (1981) The subunits of the parasporal crystal of *Bacillus thuringiensis*: size, linkage and toxicity. Arch Microbiol, **129**: 14–18.

Ignoffo CM (1973) Effects of entomopathogens on vertebrates. Ann NY Acad Sci, **217**: 141–164.

Ignoffo CM (1992) Environmental factors affecting persistence of entomopathogens. Fla Entomol, **75**: 516–525.

Innes DGL & Bendell JF (1989) The effects on small-mammal populations of aerial applications of *Bacillus thuringiensis*, fenitrothion, and Matacil® used against jack pine budworm in Ontario. Can J Zool, **67**: 1318–1323.

Jackson SG, Goodbrand RB, Ahmed R, & Kasatiya S (1995) *Bacillus cereus* and *Bacillus thuringiensis* isolated in a gastroenteritis outbreak investigation. Lett Appl Microbiol, **21**: 103–105.

Jaquet F, Hütter R, & Lüthy P (1987) Specificity of *Bacillus thuringiensis* delta-endotoxin. Appl Environ Microbiol, **53**: 500–504.

Jarrett P & Stephenson M (1990) Plasmid transfer between strains of *Bacillus thuringiensis* infecting *Galleria mellonella* and *Spodoptera littoralis*. Appl Environ Microbiol, **56**: 1608–1614.

Jensen R (1974) Comparison of various insecticides including DIPEL WP for control of the velvetbean caterpillar (*Anticarsia gemmatalis*) and the green cloverworm (*Plathypena scabra*) on soybeans and the effect on non-target species (Experiment No D911-1582). Chicago, Illinois, Abbott Laboratories Inc.

Johnson AW (1974) *Bacillus thuringiensis* and tobacco budworm control on flue-cured tobacco. J Econ Entomol, **67**: 755–759.

Juarez-Perez VM, Ferrandis MD, & Frutos R (1997) PCR-based approach for detection of novel *Bacillus thuringiensis* cry genes. Appl Environ Microbiol, **63**: 2997–3002.

Kaneko T, Nozaki R, & Aizawa K (1978) Deoxyribonucleic acid relatedness between *Bacillus anthracis*, *Bacillus cereus* and *Bacillus thuringiensis*. Microbiol Immunol, **22**: 639–641.

Kazakova SB & Dzhunusov KK (1977) The effect of Bitoxibacillin-202 on certain orchard insects in the Issyk-Kul' depression. Rev Appl Entomol, **A65**: 5987.

Keller B & Langenbruch G-A (1993) Control of coleopteran pests by *Bacillus thuringiensis*. In: Entwistle PF, Cory JS, Bailey MJ, & Higgs S ed. *Bacillus thuringiensis*, an environmental biopesticide: Theory and practice. Chichester, New York, Toronto, Wiley & Sons, pp 171–191.

Khawaled K, Ben-Dov E, Zaritsky A, & Barak Z (1990) The fate of *Bacillus thuringiensis* var. *israelensis* in *B. thuringiensis* var. *israelensis*-killed pupae of *Aedes aegypti*. J Invertebr Pathol, **56**: 312–316.

Kim HS, Lee DW, Woo SD, Yu YM, & Kang SK (1998) Seasonal distribution and characterization of *Bacillus thuringiensis* isolated from sericultural environments in Korea. J Gen Appl Microbiol, **44**: 133–138.

Klier AF & Lecadet MM (1976) Arguments based on hybridization-competition experiments in favor of the *in vitro* synthesis of sporulation-specific mRNAs by the RNA polymerase of *Bacillus thuringiensis*. Biochem Biophys Res Commun, **73**: 263–270.

Knowles BH & Ellar DJ (1987) Colloid-osmotic lysis is a general feature of the mechanisms of action of *Bacillus thuringiensis* δ-endotoxins with different insect specificity. Biochim Biophys Acta, **924**: 509–518.

Krieg A (1971) Concerning α-exotoxin produced by vegetative cells of *Bacillus thuringiensis* and *Bacillus cereus*. J Invertebr Pathol, **17**: 134–135.

Krieg A (1973) About toxic effects of cultures of *Bacillus cereus* and *Bacillus thuringiensis* on honey bees (*Apis mellifera*). Z Pflanzenkr Pflanzenschutz, **80**: 483–486.

Krieg A & Herfs W (1963) The effects of *Bacillus thuringiensis* on honey bees. Entomol Exp Appl, **6**: 1–9.

Krieg A, Hassan S, & Pinsdorf W (1980) Comparison of the effects of the variety *israelensis* with other varieties of *B. thuringiensis* on non-target organisms of the order Hymenoptera: *Trichogramma cacoeciae* and *Apis mellifera*. Anz Schädlingsk Pflanz Umweltschutz, **53**: 81–83.

Krieg A, Huger AM, Langenbruch GA, & Schnetter W (1983) *Bacillus thuringiensis* var. *tenebrionis,* a new pathotype effective against larvae of Coleoptera.. Z Angew Entomol, **96**(5): 500–508.

Krywienczyk J, Dulmage HT, & Fast PG (1978) Occurrence of two serologically distinct groups within *Bacillus thuringiensis* serotype 3ab variety *kurstaki*. J Invertebr Pathol, **37**: 372–375.

Kumar PA, Sharma RP, & Malik VS (1996) The insecticidal protein of *Bacillus thuringiensis*. Adv Appl Microbiol, **42**: 1–43.

Lacey LA & Mulla MS (1990) Safety of *Bacillus thuringiensis* ssp. *israelensis* and *Bacillus sphaericus* to nontarget organisms in the aquatic environment. In:Laird M, Lacey LA, & Davidson EW ed. Safety of microbial pesticides. Boca Raton, Florida, CRC Press, pp 169–188.

Lacey LA, Escaffre H, Philippon B, Sékétéli A, & Guillet P (1982) Large river treatment with *Bacillus thuringiensis* (H-14) for the control of *Simulium damnosum* s.l. in the Onchocerciasis Control Programme. Tropenmed Parasitol, **33**: 97–101.

Laferrière M, Bastille A, & Nadeau A (1987) Etude immunologique impliquant les composantes de l'insecticide biologique *Bacillus thuringiensis* var. *kurstaki*. St. Henri Rivière-du-Loup, Québec, Department of Public Health, Grand-Portage Regional Hospital Center, pp 1–19 (Unpublished report).

Lattin A, Grimes J, Hoxter KA, & Smith GJ (1990a) Dipel technial material (*Bacillus thuringiensis* var. *kurstaki*): An avian oral toxicity and pathogenicity study in the bobwhite (Projet No. 161-112). Easton, Maryland, Wildlife International Ltd, pp 1–25 (Unpublished Abbott document).

Lattin A, Grimes J, Hoxter K, & Smith GJ (1990b) VectoBac technical material (*Bacillus thuringiensis* var. *israelensis*): An avian oral toxicity and pathogenicity study in the malard (Project No. 161-115). Easton, Maryland, Wildlife International Ltd, pp 1–24 (Unpublished Abbott document).

Lattin A, Hoxter K, Driscoll C, Grimes J, & Jaber M (1990c) Dipel technical material (*Bacillus thuringiensis* var. *kurstaki*): An avian oral toxicity and pathogenicity study in the mallard (Project No. 161-113). Easton, Maryland, Wildlife International Ltd, pp 1–28 (Unpublished Abbott document).

Lattin A, Hoxter K, & Smith GJ (1990d) VectoBac technical material (*Bacillus thuringiensis* var. *israelensis*): An avian oral toxicity and pathogenicity study in the bobwhite (Project No. 161-114). Easton, Maryland, Wildlife International Ltd, pp 1–27 (Unpublished Abbott document).

Lechner S, Mayr R, Francis KP, Prüß BM, Kaplan T, Wießner-Gunkel E, Stewart GSAB,& Scherer S (1998) *Bacillus weihenstephanensis* sp. nov. is a new psychrotolerant species of the *Bacillus cereus* group. Int J System Bacteriol, **48**: 1373–1378.

Leong KLH, Cano RJ, & Kubinski AM (1980) Factors affecting *Bacillus thuringiensis* total field persistence. Environ Entomol, **9**: 593–599.

Levêque C, Fairhurst CP, Abbau K, Pangy D, Curtis MS, & Traoré K (1988) Onchocerciasis control programme in West Africa: ten years of monitoring fish populations. Chemosphere,**17**: 421–440.

Li J, Carroll J, & Ellar DJ (1991) Crystal structure of insecticidal (δ)-endotoxin from *Bacillus thuringiensis* at 2.5 Å resolution. Nature (Lond), **353**: 815–821.

Logan NA & Berkeley CW (1984) Identification of *Bacillus* strains using the API system. J Gen Microbiol, **130**: 1871–1882.

Lund T & Granum PE (1997) Comparison of biological effect of the two different enterotoxin complexes isolated from three different strains of *Bacillus cereus*. Microbiology, **143**: 3329–3336.

Lüthy P (1986) Insect pathogenic bacteria as pest control agents. Fortschr Zool, **32**: 201–216.

Lüthy P & Ebersold HR (1981) The entomocidal toxins of *Bacillus thuringiensis*. Pharmacol Ther, **13**: 257–283.

Lynch MJ & Baumann P (1985) Immunological comparisons of the crystal protein from strains of *Bacillus thuringiensis*. J Invertebr Pathol, **46**: 47–57.

Lynch RE, Lewis LC, & Brindley TA (1976) Bacteria associated with eggs and first-instar larvae of the European corn borer: Isolation techniques and pathogenicity. J Invertebr Pathol, **27**: 325–331.

McClintock JT, Schaffer CR, & Sjoblad RD (1995) A comparative review of the mammalian toxicity of *Bacillus thuringiensis*-based pesticides. Pestic Sci, **45**: 95–105.

Manasherob R, Ben-Dov E, Zaritsky A, & Barak Z (1998) Germination, growth, and sporulation of *Bacillus thuringiensis* subsp. *israelensis* in excreted food vacuoles of the protozoan *Tetrahymena pyriformis*. Appl Environ Microbiol, **64**: 1750–1758.

Margalit J & Dean D (1985) The story of *Bacillus thuringiensis* var. *israelensis*. J Am Mosq Control Assoc, **1**: 1–7.

Martin PAW & Travers RS (1989) Worldwide abundance and distribution of *Bacillus thuringiensis* isolates. Appl Environ Microbiol, **55**(10): 2437–2442.

Martin WF & Reichelderfer CF (1989) *Bacillus thuringiensis*: Persistence and movement in field crops. In: Abstracts of the SIP XXIInd Annual Meeting, Centre for Adult Education, University of Maryland, College Park, Maryland, 20–24 August 1989. Society for Invertebrate Pathology, p 25.

Martouret D & Euverte G (1964) The effect of *Bacillus thuringiensis* Berliner preparations on the honey bee under conditions of forced feeding. J Insect Pathol, **6**: 198–203.

Meadows MP (1993) *Bacillus thuringiensis* in the environment: Ecology and risk assessment. In: Entwistle PF, Cory JS, Bailey MJ, & Higgs S ed. *Bacillus thuringiensis*, an environmental biopesticide: Theory and practice. Chichester, New York, Toronto, Wiley & Sons, pp 193–220.

Meadows MP, Ellis DJ, Butt J, Jarrett P, & Burges HD (1992) Distribution, frequency and diversity of *Bacillus thuringiensis* in an animal feed mill. Appl Environ Microbiol, **58**(4): 1344–1350.

Melin BE & Cozzi EM (1990) Safety to nontarget invertebrates of Lepidopteran strains of *Bacillus thuringiensis* and their (ß)-exotoxins. In: Laird M, Lacey LA, & Davidson EW ed. Safety of microbial insecticides. Boca Raton, Florida, CRC Press, pp 149–167.

Menon AS & De Mestral J (1985) Survival of *Bacillus thuringiensis* var. *kurstaki* in waters. Water Air Soil Pollut, **25**: 265–274.

Merritt RW, Walker ED, Wilzbach MA, Cummins KW, & Morgan WT (1989) A broad evaluation of Bti for black fly (Diptera:Simuliidae) control in a Michigan river: efficacy, carry and nontarget effects on invertebrates and fish. J Am Mosq Control Assoc, **5**: 397–415.

Mikami T, Horikawa T, Murakami T, Sato N, Ono Y, MatsumotoT, Yamakawa A, Murayama S, Katagiri S, & Suzuki M (1995) Examination of toxin production from environmental *Bacillus cereus* and *Bacillus thuringiensis*. J Pharm Soc Jpn, **115**: 742–748.

Miura T, Takahashi RM, & Mulligan FS III (1980) Effects of the bacterial mosquito larvicide, *Bacillus thuringiensis* serotype H-14 on selected aquatic organisms. Mosq News, **40**: 619–622.

Mohd-Salleh MB, Beegle CC, & Lewis LC (1980) Fermentation media and production of exotoxin by three varieties of *Bacillus thuringiensis*. J Invertebr Pathol, **35**: 75–83.

Molloy DP (1992) Impact of the black fly (Diptera: Simuliidae) control agent *Bacillus thuringiensis* var. *israelensis* on Chironomids (Diptera: Chronomidae) and other non-target insects: results of ten field trials. J Am Mosq Control Assoc, **8**: 24–31.

Morris ON, Armstrong JA, & Hildebrand MJ (1977) Aerial field trials with a new formulation of *Bacillus thuringiensis* against the spruce budworm, *Choristoneura fumiferana* (Clem.). Ottawa, Canada, Chemical Control Research Institute (Report CC-X-144).

Morris ON, Hildebrand MJ, & Armstrong JA (1980) Preliminary field studies on the use of additives to improve deposition rate and efficacy of commercial formulations of *Bacillus thuringiensis* applied against the spruce budworm, *Choristoneura fumiferana* (Lepidoptera: Tortricidae). Sault Ste. Marie, Ontario, Canada, Forest Pest Management Institute, pp 1–23 (Report FPM-X-32).

Moulinier CL, Mas JP, Moulinier Y, De Barjac H, Giap G, &Couprie B (1995) Étude de l'innocuité de *Bacillus thuringiensis* var. *israelensis* pour les larves d'huitre. Bull Soc Pathol Exot, **74**(4): 381–391.

Mück O, Hassan S, Huger AM, & Krieg A (1981) Effects of *Bacillus thuringiensis* Berliner on the parasitic hymenoptera *Apanteles glomeratus L.* (Braconidae) and *Pimpla turionellae (L.)* (Ichneumonidiae). Z Angew Entomol, **92**: 303–314.

Mulla MS (1988) Activity, field efficacy and use of *Bacillus thuringiensis* (H-14) against mosquitoes. In: de Barjac H & Sutherland DJ ed. Bacterial control of mosquitoes and blackflies. New Brunswick, New Jersey, Rutgers University Press.

Mulla MS & Khasawinah AM (1969) Laboratory and field evaluation of larvicides against chironomid midges. J Econ Entomol, **62**: 37–41.

Mulla MS, Norland RL, Fanara DM, Darwazeh HA, & McKean DW (1971) Control of chironomid midges in recreational lakes. J Econ Entomol **64**(1): 300–307.

Mulla MS, Federici BA, & Darwazeh HA (1982) Larvicidal efficacy of*Bacillus thuringiensis* serotype H-14 against stagnant-water mosquitoes and its effects on nontarget orgnisms. Environ Entomol, **11**: 788–795.

Mulligan FS III & Schaefer CH (1982) Integration of a selective mosquito controlagent *Bacillus thuringiensis* serotype H-14, with natural predator populations in pesticidesensitive habitats. Proc Calif Mosq Vector Control Assoc, **49**: 19–22.

Murakami T, Hiraoka T, Matsumoto T, Katagiri S, Shinagawa K, &Suzuki M (1993) Analysis of common antigen of flagella in *Bacillus cereus* and *Bacillus thuringiensis*. FEMS Microbiol Lett, **107**: 179–184.

Narva KE, Payne JM, Schwab GE, Hickle LA, Galasan T, & Sick AJ (1991) Novel*Bacillus thuringiensis* microbes active against nematodes, and genes encoding novel nematode-active toxins cloned from *Bacillus thuringiensis* isolates: European patent application EP0462 721A2. Munich, Germany, European Patent Office.

Navon A (1993) Control of Lepidopteran pests with *Bacillus thuringiensis*. In: *Bacillus thuringiensis*, An Environmental Biopesticide: Theory and Practice. Eds, Entwistle PF, Cory JS, Bailey MJ & Higgs S. Chichester, New York, Toronto, Wiley & Sons, pp 126–146.

Nielsen-LeRoux C, Hansen BM, Henriksen NB (1998) Safetyof *Bacillus thuringiensis*. IOBC Bull, **21**: 269–272.

Nishikawa Y, Kramer JM, Hanaoka M, & Yasukawa A (1996) Evaluation of serotyping, biotyping, plasmid banding pattern analysis, and HEp-2 vacuolation factor assay in the epidemiological investigation of *Bacillus cereus* emetic-syndrome food poisoning. Int J Food Microbiol, **31**: 149–159.

Noble MA, Riben PD, & Cook GJ (1992) Microbiological and epidemiological surveillance programme to monitor the health effects of Foray 48B BTK spray. Vancouver, Canada, Ministry of Forests of the Province of British Columbia, pp 1–63.

Norris JR (1971) The protein crystal toxin of*Bacillus thuringiensis*: biosynthesis and physical structure. In: Burges HD & Mussey NW ed. Microbial control of insects and mites. New York, London, Academic Press Inc, pp 229–246.

Notermans S & Batt CA (1998) A risk assessment approach for food-borne *Bacillus cereus* and its toxins. J Appl Environ Microbiol Symp, **84**(suppl): 51S–61S.

Obadofin AA & Finlayson DG (1977) Interactions of several insecticides and a carabid predator (*Bembidion lampros* (Hrbst)) and their effects on *Hylemya brassicae* (Bouché). Can J Plant Sci, **57**: 1121–1126.

Ohana B, Margalit J, & Barak Z (1987) Fate of*Bacillus thuringiensis* subsp. *israelensis* under simulated field conditions. Appl Environ Microbiol, **53**: 828–831.

Ohba M & Aizawa K (1978) Serological identification of*Bacillus thuringiensis* and related bacteria isolated in Japan. J Invertebr Pathol, **32**: 303-309.

Ohba M & Aizawa K (1986) Distribution of *Bacillus thuringiensis* in soils of Japan. J Invertebr Pathol, **47**: 277–282.

Ohba M, Yu YM, & Aizawa K (1988) Occurrence of noninsecticidal *Bacillus thuringiensis* flagellar serotype 14 in the soil of Japan. Appl Microbiol, **11**: 85–89.

Olejnicek J & Maryskova B (1986), The influence of *Bacillus thuringiensis* on the mosquito predator *Notonecta glauca*. Folia Parasitol (Prague), **37**: 279.

Otvos IS & Vanderveen S (1993) Environmental report and current status of *Bacillus thuringiensis* var. *kurstaki* use for control of forest and agricultural insect pests. Victoria, British Columbia, Ministry of Forests, Forestry Canada, pp 1–81.

Pedersen JC, Damgaard PH, Eilenberg E, & Hansen BM (1995) Dispersal of *Bacillus thuringiensis* var. *kurstaki* in an experimental cabbage field. Can J Microbiol, **41**: 118–125.

Petras SF & Casida LE Jr (1985) Survival of *Bacillus thuringiensis* spores in soil. Appl Environ Microbiol, **50**: 1496–1501.

Pinnock DE, Brand RJ, Jackson KL, & Milstead JE (1974) The field persistence of *Bacillus thuringiensis* spores on *Cercis occidentalis* leaves. J Invertebr Pathol, **23**: 341–346.

Pinnock DE, Milstead JE, Kirby ME, & Nelson BJ (1977) Stability of entomopathogenic bacteria. In: Environmental stability of microbial insecticides: Miscellaneous publications. Lanham, Maryland, Entomological Society of America, vol 10, pp 77–97.

Pivovarov Yu P, Ivashina SA, & Padalkin VP (1977) [Hygienic assessment of investigation of insecticide preparations.] Gig i Sanit, **8**: 45–48 (in Russian).

Prasertphon S, Areekul P, & Tanada Y (1973) Sporulation of *Bacillus thuringiensis* in host cadavers. J Invertebr Pathol, **21**: 205–207.

Prefontaine G, Fast P, Lau PCK, Hefford MA, Hanna Z, & Brousseau R (1987) Use of oligonucleotide probes to study the relatedness of delta-endotoxin genes among *Bacillus thuringiensis* subspecies and strains. Appl Environ Microbiol, **53**: 2808–2814.

Priest FG, Goodfellow M, & Todd C (1988) A numerical classification of the genus *Bacillus*. J Gen Microbiol, **134**: 1847-1882.

Priest FG, Kaji DA, Rosato YB, & Canhos VP (1994) Characterization of *Bacillus thuringiensis* and related bacteria by ribosomal RNA gene restriction fragment length polymorphisms. Microbiology, **140**: 1015–1022.

Purcell BH (1981) Effects of *Bacillus thuringiensis* var. *israelensis* on *Aedes taeniorhynchus* and some non-target organisms in the salt marsh. Mosq News, **41**(3): 476–484.

Pusztai M, Fast P, Gringorten L, Kaplan H, Lessard T, & Carey PR (1991) The mechanism of sunlight-mediated inactivation of *Bacillus thuringiensis* crystals. Biochem J, **273**: 43–47.

Quinlan RJ (1990) Registration requirementsand safety considerations for microbial pest control agents in the European Economic Community. h: Laird M, Lacey LA, & Davidson EW ed. Safety of microbial pesticides. Boca Raton, Florida, CRC Press, pp 11–18.

Ray DE (1990) Pesticides derived from plants and other organisms In: Hayes WJ & Laws ER ed. Handbook of pesticide toxicology. New York, London, Academic Press, pp 585–636.

Reardon RC & Haissig K (1983) Spruce budworm (Lepidoptera: tortricidae) larval populations and field persistence of *Bacillus thuringiensis* after treatment in Wisconsin. J Econ Entomol,**76**: 1139–1143.

Reddy A, Battisti L, & Thorne CB (1987) Identification of self-transmissible plasmids in four *Bacillus thuringiensis* subspecies. J Bacteriol **169**(11): 5263–5270.

Rogatin AB & Baizhanov M (1984) [Laboratory study of*Bacillus thuringiensis israelensis* serotype H-14 on various groups of hydrobionts.] Izv Akad Nauk Kaz SSR Ser Biol**06**: 22–25 (in Russian).

Salama HS & Zakl FN (1983) Interaction between*Bacillus thuringiensis* Berliner and the parasites and predators of *Spodoptera littoralis* in Egypt. Z Angew Entomol, **95**: 425–429.

Salama HS, Zaki FN, & Sharaby AF (1982) Efect of *Bacillus thuringiensis* Berl. on parasites and predators of the cotton leafworm *Spodoptera littoralis* (Boisd). Z Angew Entomol, **94**: 498–504.

Saleh SM, Harris RF, & Allen ON (1970) Fate of*Bacillus thuringiensis* in soil: Effect of soil pH and organic amendment. Can J Microbiol, **16**: 677–680.

Samples JR & Buettner H (1983) Corneal ulcer caused by a biologic insecticide (*Bacillus thuringiensis*). Am J Ophthalmol, **95**(2): 258–260.

Sampson MN & Gooday GW (1998) Involvement of chitinases of*Bacillus thuringiensis* during pathogenesis in insects. Microbiology, **144**: 2189–2194.

Schnepf E, Crickmore N, van Rie J, Lereclus D, Baum J, Feitelson J, Zeigler DR, & Dean DH (1998) *Bacillus thuringiensis* and its pesticidal crystal proteins. Microbiol Mol Biol Rev,**62**: 775–806.

Schnetter W, Engler S, Morawcsik J, & Becker N (1981) [Efficacy of*Bacillus thurigiensis var. israelensis* against mosquito larvae and non-target organisms.] Mitt Dtsch Ges Allg Angew Entomol, **2**: 195–202 (in German).

Schwartz JL, Garneau L, Masson L, & Brousseau R (1991) Early response of cultured lepidopteran cells to exposure to δ-endotoxin from *Bacillus thuringiensis*: involvement of calcium and anionic channels. Biochem Biophys Acta, **1065**: 250–260.

Shadduck JA (1980) *Bacillus thuringiensis* serotype H-14 maximum challenge and eye irritation safety tests in mammals. Geneva, World Health Organization, pp 1–21 (WHO/VBC/80.763).

Shadduck JA (1983) Some considerations on the safety evaluation of nonviral microbial insecticides. WHO Bull, **6**(1): 117–128.

Sheeran W & Fisher SW (1992) The effects of agitation, sediment and competition on the persistence and efficacy of *Bacillus thuringiensis* var. *israelensis* (Bti). Ecotoxicol Environ Saf, **24**: 338–346.

Shevelev AB, Lewitin E, Novikova SI, Wojciechowska YaA, Usacheva EA, Chestukhina GG & Stepanov (1998) A new PCR-based approach to a fast search of a wide spectrum of *cry* genes from *Bacillus thuringiensis* strains. Biochem Mol Biol Int, **45**: 1265–1271.

Shinagawa K (1990) Purification and characterization of *Bacillus cereus* enterotoxin and its application to diagnosis. In: Pohland AE, Dowell VR Jr,& Richard JL ed. Microbial toxins in foods and feeds: Cellular and molecular modes of action. New York, Plenum Press, pp 181–193.

Siegel JP & Shadduck JA (1990) Clearance of *Bacillus sphaericus* and *Bacillus thuringiensis* ssp. *israelensis* from mammals. J Econ Entomol, **83**: 347–355.

Siegel JP, Shadduck JA, & Szabo J (1987) Safety of the entomopathogen *Bacillus thuringiensis* var. *israelensis* for mammals. J Econ Entomol, **80**: 717–723.

Slatin SL, Abrams CK, & English L (1990) Delta-endotoxins form cation-selective channels in planar lipid bilayers. Biochem Biophys Res Commun, **169**: 765–772.

Slepecky RA & Hemphill HE (1992) The genus *Bacillus*-nonmedical. In: Balows A, Truper HG, Dworkin M, Harder W, & Schleifer K-H ed. The prokaryotes, 2nd ed. New York, Basel, Springer-Verlag, vol II, pp 1663–1696.

Smedley DP & Ellar DJ (1996) Mutagenesis of 3 surface-exposed loops of a *Bacillus thuringiensis* insecticidal toxin reveals residues important for toxicity, recognition and possibly membrane insertion. Microbiology, **142**: 1617–1624.

Smith RA (1987) Use of crystal serology to differentiate among varieties of *Bacillus thuringiensis*. J Invertebr Pathol, **50**: 1–8.

Smith RA & Couche GA (1991) The phylloplane as a source of *Bacillus thuringiensis* variants. Appl Environ Microbiol, **57**: 311–315.

Snarski VM (1990) Interactions between *Bacillus thuringiensis* subsp. *israelensis* and fathead minnows, *Pimephales promelas* Rafinesque, under laboratory conditions. Appl Environ Microbiol, **56**: 2618–2622.

Sorenson AA & Falcon LA (1980) Comparison of microdroplet and high volume application of *Bacillus thuringiensis* on pear suppression of fruit tree leaf roller *Acrhips argyrospilus* and coverage on foliage and fruit. Environ Entomol, **9**: 350.

Stahly DP, Dingman DW, Bulla LA Jr, & Aronson AI (1978) Possible origin and function of the parasporal crystals in *Bacillus thuringiensis*. Biochem Biophys Res Commun, **84**(3): 581–588.

Stahly DP, Andrews RE, & Yousten AA (1991) The genus *Bacillus*-insect pathogens. In: Balows A, Truper HG, Dworkin M, Harder W, & Schleifer K-H ed. The prokaryotes, 2nd ed. New York, Basel, Springer-Verlag, vol II, pp 1697–1745.

Surprenant DC (1989) Acute toxicity of *Bacillus thuringiensis* var. *tenebrionis* technical material to rainbow trout (*Salmo gairdneri*) under static renewal conditions. Wareham, Massachusetts, Springborn Life Sciences Inc., pp 1–19 (Unpublished Abbott document).

Tayabali AF & Seligy VL (1997) Cell integrity markers for *in vitro* evaluation of cytotoxic responses to bacteria-containing commercial insecticides. Ecotoxicol Environ Saf, **37**: 152–162.

Thomas WE & Ellar DJ (1983) *Bacillus thuringiensis* var. *israelensis* crystal δ-endotoxin: effects on insect and mammalian cells *in vitro* and *in vivo*. J Cell Sci, **60**: 181–197.

Thomas EM & Watson TF (1986) Effect of Dipel (*Bacillus thuringiensis*) on the survival of immature and adult *Hyposoter exiguae* (Hymenoptera: Ichneumonidae). J Invertebr Pathol, **47**: 178–183.

Tomlin CDS ed. (1997) The pesticide manual, 11th ed. Farnham, Surrey, British Crop Protection Council, 1606 pp.

Travers RS, Martin PAW, & Reichelderfer CF (1987) Selective process for efficient isolation of soil *Bacillus* spp. Appl Environ Microbiol, **53**: 1263–1266.

Väisänen OM, Mwaisumo NJ, & Salkinoja-Salonen MS (1991) Differentiation of dairy strains of the *Bacillus cereus* group by phage typing, minimum growth temperature, and fatty acid analysis. J Appl Bacteriol, **70**: 315-324.

Van Frankenhuyzen K (1993) The challenge of *Bacillus thuringiensis*. In: Entwistle PF, Cory JS, Bailey MJ, & Higgs S ed. *Bacillus thuringiensis*, an environmental biopesticide: Theory and practice. Chichester, New York, Toronto, Wiley & Sons, pp 1–35.

Vaòková J & Purrini K (1979) Natural epizooties caused by bacilli of the species *Bacillus thuringiensis* and *Bacillus cereus*. Z Angew Entomol, **88**: 216–221.

Van Rie J, Jansens S, Höfte H, Degheele D, & Van Mellaert H (1989), Specificity of *Bacillus thuringiensis* δ-endotoxins: Importance of specific receptors on the brush border membrane of the mid-gut of target insects. Eur J Biochem, **186**: 239–247.

Venkateswerlu G & Stotzky G (1992) Binding of the protoxin and toxin proteins of *Bacillus thuringiensis* subsp. *kurstaki* on clay minerals. Curr Microbiol, **25**: 225–233.

Visser B, Bosch D, & Honée G (1993) Domain-function studies of *Bacillus thuringiensis* crystal proteins: a genetic approach. In: Entwistle PF, Cory JS, Bailey MJ, & Higgs S ed. *Bacillus thuringiensis*, an environmental piopesticide: Theory and practice. Chichester, New York, Toronto, Wiley & Sons, pp 71–88.

Wallner W & Surgeoner G (1974) Control of oakleaf caterpillar, *Heterocampa manteo*, and the impact of controls on nontarget organisms. Chicago, Illinois, Abbott Laboratories (Unpublished document).

Wallner WE, Dubois NR, & Grinberg PS (1983) Alteration of parasitism by *Rogas lymantriae* (Hymenoptera: Braconidae) in *Bacillus thuringiensis*-stressed gypsy moth (Lepidoptera: Lymantriidae) hosts. J Econ Entomol, **76**: 275–277.

Warren RE, Rubenstein D, Ellar DJ, Kramer JM, & Gilbert RJ (1984) *Bacillus thuringiensis* var. *israelensis*: Protoxin activation and safety. Lancet: **March 24**: 678–679.

Weires RW & Smith GL (1977) Apple mite control. Hudson Valley, New York, New York State Agricultural Experimental Station.

Weseloh RM & Andreadis TG (1982) Possible mechanism for synergism between *Bacillus thuringiensis* and the gypsy moth (Lepidoptera: Lymantriidae) parasitoid, *Apanteles melanoscelus* (Hymenoptera: Braconidae). Ann Entomol Soc Am, **75**: 435–438.

Weseloh RM, Andreadis TG, Moore REB, & Anderson JF (1983) Field confirmation of a mechanism causing synergism between *Bacillus thuringiensis* and the gypsy moth parasitoid, *Apanteles melanoscelus*. J Invertebr Pathol, **41**: 99–103.

West AW, Burges HD, & Wyborn CH (1984a) Effect of incubation in natural and autoclaved soil upon potency and viability of *Bacillus thuringiensis*. J Invertebr Pathol, **44**: 121–127.

West AW, Burges HD, White JR, & Wyborn CH (1984b) Persistence of *Bacillus thuringiensis* parasporal crystal insecticidal activity in soil. J Invertebr Pathol, **44**: 128–133.

WHO (1982) Data sheet on the biological control agent *Bacillus thuringiensis* serotype H-14 (de Barjac 1978). Geneva, World Health Organization (WHO/VBC/79.750 Rev. 1).

WHO (1985) Ninth report of the WHO Expert Committee on Vector Biology and Control — Safe Use of Pesticides. Geneva, World Health Organization (WHO Technical Report Series No. 720).

WHO (1991) Fourteenth report of the WHO Expert Committee on Vector Biology and Control — Safe Use of Pestidides. Geneva, World Health Organization (WHO Technical Report Series No. 813).

Wilkinson JD, Biever KD, & Ignoffo CM (1975) Contact toxicity of some chemical and biological pesticides to several insect parasitoids and predators. Entomophaga, **20**: 113–120.

Workman RB (1977) Pesticides toxic to striped earwig, an important insect predator. Proc Fla State Hortic Soc, **90**: 401–402.

Wunschel D, Fox KF, Black GE, & Fox A (1994) Discrimination among the *B. cereus* group, in comparison to *B. subtilis*, by structural carbohydrate profiles and ribosomal RNA spacer region PCR. System Appl Microbiol, **17**: 625–635.

Yameogo L, Levêque C, Traoré K, & Fairhurst CP (1988) Dix ans de surveillance de la faune aquatique des rivières d'Afrique de l'Ouest traitées contre les Simulides (Diptera: Simuliidae), agents vecteurs de l'onchocercose humaine. Nat Can, **115**: 287–298.

Yousten AA (1973) Effect of the *Bacillus thuringiensis* δ-endotoxin on an insect predator which has consumed intoxicated cabbage looper larvae. J Invertebr Pathol, **21**: 312–314.

Yousten AA, Genthner FJ, & Benfield EF (1992) Fate of *Bacillus sphaericus* and *Bacillus thuringiensis* serovar *israelensis* in the aquatic environment. J Am Mosq Control Assoc, **8**: 143–148.

Zahner V, Momen H, Salles CA, & Rabinovitch L (1989) A comparative study of enzyme variation in *Bacillus cereus* and *Bacillus thuringiensis*. J Appl Bacteriol, **67**: 275-282.

Zukowski K (1995) [Laboratory examination of the effectiveness of new biological preparations for reducing populations of cockroaches (*Blattella germanica* L.)]. Rocz Panstw Zakl Hig, **46**: 293–297 (in Polish).

RÉSUMÉ

La présente monographie traite des agents microbiens de lutte contre les nuisibles utilisant le bacille *Bacillus thuringiensis* (Bt). Ce bacille, qui est aussi appelé bacille de Thuringe, est également une source très importante de gènes utilisée pour conférer aux plantes et aux microorganismes transgéniques (ou organismes génétiquement modifiés, *OGM*) la faculté de résister aux ravageurs et autres nuisibles. Les effets que pourraient avoir ces OGM sur la santé humaine et l'environnement présentent divers aspects qui sont sans rapport ou tout au plus en rapport lointain avec les produits à base de Bt et n'entrent pas, par conséquent, dans le cadre de la présente monographie.

1. Identité, caractéristiques biologiques et méthodes d'analyse

Bacillus thuringiensis est une bactérie anaérobie facultative, gram-positif, qui forme des inclusions protéiques caractéristiques adjacentes à l'endosporc. Certaines sous-espèces de Bt peuvent synthétiser plusieurs inclusions parasporales. Le Bt est génétiquement indiscernable du Bc, exception faite de son aptitude à former des inclusions cristallines parasporales qui sont toxiques pour certains invertébrés, notamment les larves d'insectes appartenant aux ordres suivants: coléoptères, diptères et lépidoptères. Les inclusions parasporales sont constituées de diverses protéines cristallisées insecticides (ICP). Ces cristaux sont de forme variable (bipyramidale, cuboïdale, rhomboïdale plane, sphérique ou composite, c'est-à-dire comportant deux types de cristaux) selon la nature des protéines qui les composent. On a établi une corrélation partielle entre la morphologie des cristaux, la composition en protéines cristallisées et l'activité biologique vis-à-vis des insectes.

Le taxon phénotypique fondamental est la sous-espèce, caractérisée par son sérotype flagellaire (H). En 1998, on avait déjà décrit 67 sous-espèces. Les gènes qui codent pour les ICP sont pour la plupart situés sur les plasmides. Chacune de ces protéines n'est le produit que d'un seul gène. La plupart des plasmides porteurs de gènes ICP se transmettent facilement d'une souche bactérienne à l'autre par conjugaison et peuvent aussi passer à une espèce bactérienne voisine.

La classification phénotypique est maintenant complétée par une caractérisation basée sur la biologie moléculaire et plus précisément sur la séquence des gènes codant pour les cristaux (*cry* et *cyt*) plutôt que sur la spécificité vis-à-vis des insectes cibles. Divers domaines des ICP sont responsables de la sensibilité de l'hôte (reconnaissance des récepteurs) et de la toxicité (formation de pores).

Parmi les techniques couramment utilisées pour caractériser les souches de Bt ou les inclusions protéiques elles-mêmes, on peut citer l'analyse des acides gras pariétaux, les anticorps monoclonaux, les sondes d'ADN oligonucléotidiques, les profils plasmidiques, l'analyse par amplification génique (PCR), la technique des empreintes génétiques et les profils électrophorétiques SDS-PAGE (électrophorèse en gel de polyacrylamide en présence de dodécylsulfate de sodium).

Certaines sous-espèces de Bt produisent pendant leur croissance une bêta-exotoxine constitué d'un nucléotide thermostable qui peut contaminer les produits. Cette bêta-exotoxine est toxique pour presque toutes les formes de vie, y compris l'Homme et les insectes cibles. Au cours de leur croissance, les diverses souches de Bt produisent toutes sortes d'antibiotiques, d'enzymes, de métabolites et de toxines, y compris des toxines Bc, qui peuvent avoir des effets nocifs sur les organismes visés ou non visés. La numération des spores n'est pas le reflet fidèle de l'activité insecticide d'une souche de Bt ou d'un produit qui en dérive. Pour mesurer l'activité (en unités toxicologiques internationales (ITU) par mg), on procède à un test biologique sur insecte au moyen d'un étalon international.

2. Mode d'action sur les insectes cibles

Les Bt sporulés ou les complexes spores-ICP doivent être ingérés par les larves d'insectes appartenant aux espèces sensibles. L'efficacité des ICP dépend de plusieurs facteurs: solubilisation dans l'intestin moyen, conversion de la protoxine en toxine biologiquement active sous l'action des enzymes protéolytiques, fixation de la toxine active aux récepteurs membranaires spécifiques par sa région C-terminale et formation de pores par la région N-terminale entraînant la lyse des cellules épithéliales. La germination des spores et la prolifération de cellules bactériennes végétatives dans l'hémocèle peut entraîner une septicémie qui contribue également à la mort. La spécificité d'hôte des différentes ICP est essentiellement déterminée par leur fixation aux récepteurs.

3. Habitats

On a isolé de nombreuses sous-espèces de Bt sur des insectes morts ou mourants appartenant principalement à l'ordre des coléoptères, des diptères et des lépidoptères, mais nombreuses sont également celles qui ont été isolées du sol, de la surface des feuilles ou d'autres habitats. Les cadavres d'insectes contiennent souvent de grandes quantités de spores et d'ICP susceptibles de pénétrer dans l'environnement. Les sous-espèces actives contre les coléoptères et les lépidoptères sont principalement associées au sol et aux surfaces foliaires, alors que les sous-espèces actives contre les diptères se rencontrent communément dans les milieux aquatiques. Dans l'environnement, les spores sont capables de persister et de se développer en présence de conditions favorables et de nutriments appropriés.

4. Produits du commerce. Production et épandage

Les produits commerciaux classiques à base de bacille de Thuringe, qui utilisent des souches naturelles, représentent environ 90% du marché mondial des agents microbiologiques de lutte contre les nuisibles. La plupart de ces produits contiennent des spores viables et des ICP, mais dans certains d'entre eux, les spores sont inactivées (Bti). Chaque année, on en produit quelque 13 000 tonnes par la technique de fermentation aérobie. Les produits classiques à base de Bt sont principalement destinés à lutter contre les lépidoptères qui ravagent les cultures et les plantations forestières; toutefois, ces dernières années, on a également commercialisé des souches actives contre les coléoptères. Les programmes de santé publique utilisent également des souches de Bti actives contre les diptères vecteurs de maladies virales ou parasitaires.

Les formulations commerciales de bacille de Thuringe peuvent être épandues sur le feuillage, le sol, les étendues d'eaux ou dans les entrepôts de denrées alimentaires pour combattre les insectes. Une fois le produit épandu dans l'écosystème, les cellules bactériennes végétatives et les spores peuvent persister à des concentrations progressivement décroissantes pendant des semaines, des mois ou des années en tant que constituants de la microflore naturelle. Par contre, les ICP perdent leur activité biologique au bout de quelques heures ou de quelques jours.

5. Effets du Bt sur les organismes non visés

Les études effectuées sur des mammifères et notamment celles qui ont porté sur des animaux de laboratoire ont consisté a évaluer l'infectiosité et la toxicité éventuelles de diverses préparations à base de Bt contenant notamment des ICP, des spores et des cellules bactériennes en phase végétative. Sous ces trois formes, les différentes sous-espèces de Bt se sont révélées pour la plupart non pathogènes et non toxiques pour les diverses espèces animales utilisées. On a montré que les cellules bactériennes en phase végétative et les spores persistaient pendant plusieurs semaines sans causer d'effets nocifs. En particulier, on a constaté que le Bt n'avait pas d'effets indésirables sur les oiseaux, les poissons et de nombreux autres vertébrés aquatiques non visés, lors d'études en laboratoire ou sur le terrain portant sur un grand nombre de spécimens. Il n'y a que relativement peu d'invertébrés aquatiques qui se révèlent sensibles au Bt en laboratoire ou sur le terrain. Par ailleurs, le bacille de Thuringe n'exerce pas non plus d'effets nocifs sur les lombrics.

L'activité insecticide des différentes sous-espèces de Bt présente en général une spécificité d'hôte très marquée vis-à-vis des coléoptères, des diptères et des lépidoptères et on a montré qu'elle n'avait pratiquement aucun effet toxique direct sur les arthropodes non visés. La plupart des données relatives à l'innocuité de ces produits pour les arthropodes non visés concernent les sous-espèces de Bt actives contre les diptères et les lépidoptères.

Les études consacrées aux formulations de Bti exemptes de contaminants toxiques ont montré qu'elles étaient sans danger pour la plupart des arthropodes non visés. Certains moucherons (chironomides appartenant à l'ordre des diptères) très proches des moustiques se sont révélés sensibles à de fortes doses de Bti mais ne sont nullement affectés aux doses utilisées pour la destruction des larves de moustiques. Des études sur le terrain ont mis en évidence des cas de réduction ou au contraire d'augmentation de certaines populations d'arthropodes non visés.

Les études toxicologiques auxquelles ont été soumis de nombreux ordres d'insectes n'ont, pour la plupart d'entre eux, révélé aucun effet toxique imputable au Btk.

On a observé une certaine mortalité chez des abeilles (*Apis mellifera*) qui avaient été soumises à des bacilles des sous-espèces Btt et Btk en phase végétative, mais il ne semble pas que les spores ou les ICP soient capables de produire un tel effet. En laboratoire et sur le terrain, le Btg n'a aucun effet toxique sur les abeilles.

Les souches de Bte productrices de bêta-exotoxine se sont révélées capables d'exercer des effets toxiques sur les arthropodes non visés.

6. Exposition humaine et effets du bacille de Thuringe sur l'Homme

Les ouvriers qui épandent des produits à base de Bt peuvent être fortement exposés à ces produits par contact cutané ou par inhalation d'aérosols. L'usage du Bt en agriculture peut entraîner la contamination de l'eau potable et des denrées alimentaires par le bacille. Toutefois, à l'exception de quelques cas d'irritation des yeux ou de la peau, on n'a pas connaissance d'effets nocifs attestés qui résulteraient d'une exposition professionnelle à des produits à base de Bt. Des volontaires qui avaient ingéré ou inhalé de grandes quantités de diverses formulations de Btk, n'ont ressenti aucun effet indésirable. On a mis en évidence des anticorps dirigés contre les cellules bactériennes, les spores et les complexes spores-cristaux chez des ouvriers chargés de l'épandage de produits à base de Bt; aucun effet indésirable n'a cependant été observé. On connaît le cas d'un certain nombre de patients atteints de maladies infectieuses chez lesquels la présence de Bt a été mise en évidence. Toutefois, aucune des études qui leur ont été consacrées n'a permis de conclure de façon certaine que l'utilisation du Bt comporte effectivement un risque pour la santé humaine. Il ne semble pas non plus que la présence de Bt dans l'eau destinée à la consommation ou dans les denrées alimentaires soit à l'origine d'effets indésirables chez l'Homme.

7. Conclusions

Compte tenu de la spécificité de leur mode d'action, il est improbable que les produits à base de Bt constituent un danger quelconque pour l'Homme et les vertébrés ni pour la très grande majorité des invertébrés non visés, pour autant qu'ils ne contiennent pas d'autres microorganismes ou de substances biologiquement actives autres que les ICP. On peut utiliser ces produits en toute sécurité pour détruire les insectes qui ravagent les domaines agricoles et horticoles ainsi que les forêts. Ils sont également sans danger pour le milieu aquatique et on peut notamment les épandre dans les réservoirs d'eau potable pour lutter contre les moustiques, les simulies et les larves d'insectes incommodants. Il convient cependant de noter qu'en phase végétative, le Bt est capable de produire des toxines de type Bc dont on ignore si elles sont susceptibles de provoquer des maladies chez l'Homme.

1. RESUMEN

Esta monografía trata sobre los plaguicidas microbianos (PM) basados en *Bacillus thuringiensis* (Bt). Esta bacteria es también una fuente clave de genes cuya expresión transgénica confiere resistencia frente a plagas a plantas y microorganismos, actuando como plaguicida en los denominados organismos modificados genéticamente (OMG). Los posibles efectos de los OMG sobre la salud humana y el medio están poco o nada relacionados con los productos basados en Bt, por lo que quedan fuera del ámbito de esta monografía.

1. Identidad, características biológicas y métodos de laboratorio

Bt es una bacteria gram-positiva y anaerobia facultativa que forma inclusiones proteicas características junto a la endospora. Las subespecies de Bt pueden sintetizar más de una inclusión parasporal. Desde el punto de vista genético, Bt es indistinguible de Bc, exceptuando la capacidad de Bt para producir inclusiones parasporales cristalinas que son tóxicas para ciertos invertebrados, en particular para las larvas de insectos pertenecientes a los órdenes *Coleóptera*, *Díptera* y *Lepidóptera*. Dichas inclusiones parasporales están formadas por distintas proteínas cristalinas insecticidas (PCI). Los cristales tienen formas diversas (bipiramidales, cuboides, romboides planos, esféricos o compuestos por dos tipos de cristales), dependiendo de su composición en PCI. Se ha comprobado que existe una correlación parcial entre la morfología del cristal, la composición en PCI y la bioactividad frente a los insectos diana.

El taxón fenotípico básico es la subespecie, identificada por el serotipo flagelar (H). Hasta 1998 se habían descrito 67 subespecies. Los genes que codifican las PCI se encuentran fundamentalmente en los plásmidos. Cada PCI es el producto de un solo gen. La mayoría de los plásmidos con genes de PCI se transfieren fácilmente por conjugación entre cepas de Bt y pueden transferirse a especies bacterianas emparentadas. La clasificación fenotípica se ha complementado en la actualidad con la caracterización biomolecular, basada en la secuencia de los genes de las proteínas cristalinas (*cry* y *cyt*), no en la especificidad para las especies diana. En las PCI, la susceptibilidad del huésped (reconocimiento de receptores) y la toxicidad (formación de poros) son responsabilidad de dominios distintos de la molécula.

Las técnicas utilizadas habitualmente para caracterizar las cepas de Bt o la propia PCI consisten en análisis de los ácidos grasos de la pared celular, anticuerpos monoclonales, sondas de oligonucleótidos de ADN, perfiles de plásmidos, análisis por reacción en cadena de la polimerasa (PCR), estudios del ADN (huella genética) y perfiles de SDS-PAGE (dodecil sulfato sódico — electroforesis en gel de poliacrilamida).

La beta-exotoxina, un nucleótido termoestable, es sintetizada por algunas subespecies de Bt durante el crecimiento vegetativo y puede contaminar los productos. Es tóxica para casi todas las formas de vida, incluidos los seres humanos y los órdenes de insectos diana. Durante el crecimiento vegetativo, varias cepas de Bt producen una gama de antibióticos, enzimas, metabolitos y toxinas, incluidas toxinas de Bc, que pueden tener efectos nocivos tanto en las especies que son objetivo del plaguicida como en las que no lo son. Los recuentos de esporas no reflejan con exactitud la actividad insecticida de una cepa o un preparado de Bt. Se mide la potencia (UTI/mg) de cada producto mediante ensayos biológicos para los que se utiliza un patrón internacional basado en un insecto concreto.

2. Modo de acción en los insectos diana

Es preciso que las larvas de los insectos susceptibles ingieran Bt esporulado con PCI o con complejos espora-PCI. La eficacia de la PCI depende de su solubilización en el intestino medio, de la conversión de la protoxina en la toxina biológicamente activa por la acción de enzimas proteolíticas, de la unión específica del dominio C-terminal de la toxina activa al receptor de membrana y de la formación de poros por parte del dominio N-terminal, con la consiguiente lisis de las células epiteliales. La germinación de esporas y la proliferación de células vegetativas en el hemocele puede ocasionar una septicemia y contribuir a la muerte. La unión de la PCI al receptor es el determinante principal de la especificidad de huésped para las distintas PCI de Bt.

3. Hábitats

Se han aislado muchas subespecies de Bt a partir de insectos muertos o moribundos, la mayoría pertenecientes a los órdenes *Coleóptera*, *Díptera* y *Lepidóptera*, pero también del suelo, de superficies foliares y de otros hábitats. Los exoesqueletos de insectos muertos contienen a menudo grandes cantidades de esporas y PCI que pueden incorporarse al medio. Las subespecies de Bt activas frente a coleópteros y lepidópteros se asocian fundamentalmente con el suelo y el filoplano (superficies foliares), mientras que las activas frente a dípteros se hallan generalmente en medios acuáticos. En el ambiente, las esporas persisten y pueden entrar en crecimiento vegetativo cuando las condiciones son favorables y hay nutrientes disponibles.

4. Productos comerciales, producción y aplicación

Los preparados convencionales de Bt, que utilizan cepas de Bt que aparecen de forma espontánea en la naturaleza, representan aproximadamente el 90% del mercado mundial de los PM. La mayoría de los preparados de Bt contienen PCI y esporas viables, pero en algunos productos de Bti las esporas están inactivadas. Cada año se producen aproximadamente 13.000 toneladas utilizando tecnología de fermentación aerobia. Los preparados convencionales de Bt tienen como objetivos primarios las plagas de lepidópteros que afectan a los cultivos agrícolas y forestales; sin embargo, en los últimos años también se han comercializado cepas de Bt activas frente a plagas de coleópteros. Se están utilizando en programas de salud pública cepas de Bti activas frente a dípteros vectores de enfermedades parasitarias y víricas.

Las formulaciones comerciales de Bt pueden aplicarse como insecticidas al follaje, el suelo, el medio acuático o instalaciones de almacenamiento de alimentos. Tras aplicar una subespecie de Bt a un ecosistema, las células vegetativas y las esporas pueden persistir en concentraciones gradualmente decrecientes durante semanas, meses o años como un componente de la microflora natural. Sin embargo, las PCI pierden su actividad biológica en horas o días.

5. Efectos de Bt sobre especies que no son objetivo del plaguicida

En estudios con mamíferos, en particular con animales de laboratorio, se ha evaluado la posible infecciosidad y toxicidad de diversos preparados de Bt, que comprenden las PCI, células vegetativas y esporas. Las PCI, las esporas y las células vegetativas de las subespecies de Bt, que se administraron por distintas vías, carecían en su mayoría de patogenicidad y toxicidad para las diversas especies animales estudiadas. Se comprobó que las células vegetativas o las esporas de Bt persistían durante semanas sin causar efectos adversos. No se ha observado que Bt afecte a pájaros, peces o muchas otras especies de vertebrados acuáticos que no son objetivo del plaguicida y se han estudiado en gran número de trabajos de laboratorio y de campo. Son relativamente pocas las especies de invertebrados acuáticos susceptibles a Bt, tanto en condiciones de laboratorio como de campo. Bt no afecta a las lombrices de tierra.

En general, las subespecies de Bt muestran gran especificidad en su actividad insecticida frente a *Coleóptera*, *Díptera* y *Lepidóptera,* así como una toxicidad directa escasa, si no nula, frente a los artrópodos que no son su objetivo. La mayor parte de los datos disponibles sobre inocuidad en éstos se han obtenido con las subespecies de Bt activas frente a *Díptera* y *Lepidóptera*.

Los estudios sobre formulaciones de Bti sin contaminantes tóxicos no han puesto de manifiesto efectos nocivos en la gran mayoría de los artrópodos que no son objetivo del plaguicida. Se ha comprobado que algunas moscas enanas (*Díptera*: *Chironomidae*), estrechamente emparentadas con los mosquitos, son sensibles a dosis altas de Bti, pero no se ven afectadas por dosis letales para larvas de mosquito. En estudios de campo se han descrito disminuciones o aumentos transitorios de las poblaciones de algunos artrópodos que no son objetivo del plaguicida.

Se han estudiado muchos órdenes de insectos, tanto en el laboratorio como en trabajos de campo, y se ha comprobado que en la mayoría de ellos Btk no tiene efecto.

Se ha observado mortalidad en abejas melíferas (*Apis mellifera*) tras la exposición a Btt y Btk en crecimiento vegetativo, pero el efecto no parece guardar relación con las esporas o las PCI. En los estudios de laboratorio y de campo, Btg no mostró efectos adversos sobre las abejas melíferas.

Se ha comprobado que cepas de Bte productoras de beta-exotoxina tienen efectos adversos sobre artrópodos que no son objetivo del plaguicida.

6. Exposición a Bt y efectos sobre los seres humanos

La aplicación agrícola de preparados de Bt puede suponer una considerable exposición de los trabajadores, tanto en aerosol como dérmica. Puede, asimismo, causar la contaminación del agua potable y los alimentos por la bacteria. Salvo casos notificados de irritación ocular y dérmica, no se han documentado efectos adversos sobre la salud tras la exposición laboral a preparados de Bt. Individuos voluntarios ingirieron e inhalaron grandes cantidades de una formulación de Btk sin sufrir efectos adversos. Se detectaron títulos de anticuerpos frente a las células vegetativas, las esporas y los complejos espora-cristal en trabajadores que pulverizaban preparados de Bt, pero no se registraron efectos adversos. Se han descrito algunos casos de presencia de Bt en pacientes con diversas enfermedades infecciosas. Sin embargo, ninguno de estos estudios demuestra de forma inequívoca que el uso de Bt entrañe un riesgo real para la salud humana. No se ha demostrado que Bt tenga efectos adversos en seres humanos cuando está presente en el agua potable o los alimentos.

7. Conclusiones

Debido a la especificidad de su modo de acción, es improbable que los preparados de Bt entrañen peligro alguno para los seres humanos u otros vertebrados, o para la gran mayoría de los invertebrados que no constituyen su objetivo, siempre y cuando no contengan microorganismos distintos de Bt y productos biológicamente activos distintos de las PCI. Los preparados de Bt pueden utilizarse con seguridad para controlar las plagas de insectos de los cultivos agrícolas y hortícolas, así como las forestales. También es seguro su uso en medios acuáticos, incluidos los depósitos de agua potable, para controlar el mosquito, la mosca negra y las larvas de insectos dañinos. Sin embargo, es preciso señalar que las formas vegetativas de Bt pueden sintetizar toxinas del tipo de las producidas por Bc, cuya importancia como causa de enfermedades humanas se desconoce.

Food additives and contaminants in food, principles for the safety assessment of (No. 70, 1987)
Formaldehyde (No. 89, 1989)
Genetic effects in human populations, guidelines for the study of (No. 46, 1985)
Glyphosate (No. 159, 1994)
Guidance values for human exposure limits (No. 170, 1994)
Heptachlor (No. 38, 1984)
Hexachlorobenzene (No. 195, 1997)
Hexachlorobutadiene (No. 156, 1994)
Alpha- and beta-hexachlorocyclohexanes (No. 123, 1992)
Hexachlorocyclopentadiene (No. 120, 1991)
n-Hexane (No. 122, 1991)
Human exposure assessment (No. 214, 1999)
Hydrazine (No. 68, 1987)
Hydrogen sulfide (No. 19, 1981)
Hydroquinone (No. 157, 1994)
Immunotoxicity associated with exposure to chemicals, principles and methods for assessment (No. 180, 1996)
Infancy and early childhood, principles for evaluating health risks from chemicals during (No. 59, 1986)
Isobenzan (No. 129, 1991)
Isophorone (No. 174, 1995)
Kelevan (No. 66, 1986)
Lasers and optical radiation (No. 23, 1982)
Lead (No. 3, 1977)[a]
Lead, inorganic (No. 165, 1995)
Lead – environmental aspects (No. 85, 1989)
Lindane (No. 124, 1991)
Linear alkylbenzene sulfonates and related compounds (No. 169, 1996)
Magnetic fields (No. 69, 1987)
Man-made mineral fibres (No. 77, 1988)
Manganese (No. 17, 1981)
Mercury (No. 1, 1976)[a]
Mercury – environmental aspects (No. 86, 1989)
Mercury, inorganic (No. 118, 1991)
Methanol (No. 196, 1997)
Methomyl (No. 178, 1996)
2-Methoxyethanol, 2-ethoxyethanol, and their acetates (No. 115, 1990)
Methyl bromide (No. 166, 1995)
Methylene chloride
(No. 32, 1984, 1st edition)
(No. 164, 1996, 2nd edition)
Methyl ethyl ketone (No. 143, 1992)
Methyl isobutyl ketone (No. 117, 1990)
Methylmercury (No. 101, 1990)
Methyl parathion (No. 145, 1992)
Methyl *tertiary*-butyl ether (No. 206, 1998)
Mirex (No. 44, 1984)
Morpholine (No. 179, 1996)
Mutagenic and carcinogenic chemicals, guide to short-term tests for detecting (No. 51, 1985)
Mycotoxins (No. 11, 1979)
Mycotoxins, selected: ochratoxins, trichothecenes, ergot (No. 105, 1990)
Nephrotoxicity associated with exposure to chemicals, principles and methods for the assessment of (No. 119, 1991)
Neurotoxicity associated with exposure to chemicals, principles and methods for the assessment of (No. 60, 1986)
Nickel (No. 108, 1991)
Nitrates, nitrites, and *N*-nitroso compounds (No. 5, 1978)[a]
Nitrogen oxides
(No. 4, 1977, 1st edition)[a]
(No. 188, 1997, 2nd edition)
2-Nitropropane (No. 138, 1992)
Noise (No. 12, 1980)[a]
Organophosphorus insecticides: a general introduction (No. 63, 1986)
Paraquat and diquat (No. 39, 1984)
Pentachlorophenol (No. 71, 1987)
Permethrin (No. 94, 1990)
Pesticide residues in food, principles for the toxicological assessment of (No. 104, 1990)
Petroleum products, selected (No. 20, 1982)
Phenol (No. 161, 1994)
d-Phenothrin (No. 96, 1990)
Phosgene (No. 193, 1997)
Phosphine and selected metal phosphides (No. 73, 1988)
Photochemical oxidants (No. 7, 1978)
Platinum (No. 125, 1991)
Polybrominated biphenyls (No. 152, 1994)
Polybrominated dibenzo-*p*-dioxins and dibenzofurans (No. 205, 1998)
Polychlorinated biphenyls and terphenyls
(No. 2, 1976, 1st edition)[a]
(No. 140, 1992, 2nd edition)
Polychlorinated dibenzo-*p*-dioxins and dibenzofurans (No. 88, 1989)
Polycyclic aromatic hydrocarbons, selected non-heterocyclic (No. 202, 1998)
Progeny, principles for evaluating health risks associated with exposure to chemicals during pregnancy (No. 30, 1984)
1-Propanol (No. 102, 1990)
2-Propanol (No. 103, 1990)
Propachlor (No. 147, 1993)
Propylene oxide (No. 56, 1985)
Pyrrolizidine alkaloids (No. 80, 1988)
Quintozene (No. 41, 1984)
Quality management for chemical safety testing (No. 141, 1992)
Radiofrequency and microwaves (No. 16, 1981)
Radionuclides, selected (No. 25, 1983)
Resmethrins (No. 92, 1989)

---

[a] Out of print